OBSTETRICS

MEDICAL SCHOOL CRASH COURSE

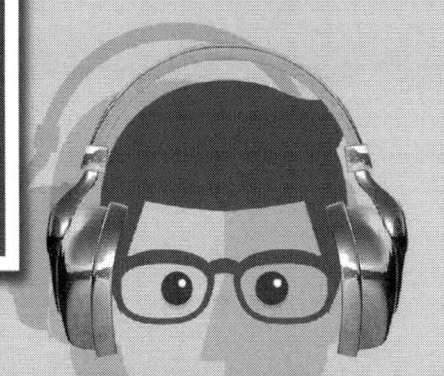

HIGH-YIELD CONTENT REVIEW
Q&A AND "KEY TAKEAWAYS"
TOP 100 TEST QUESTIONS

FOLLOW-ALONG PDF MANUAL

audiolearn

audiolearn

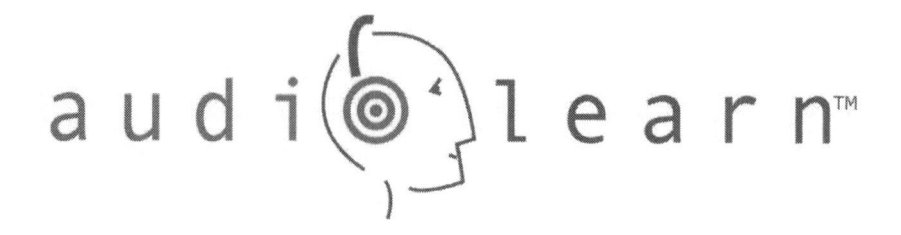

OBSTETRICS

Medical School Crash Course™

www.AudioLearn.com

Table of Contents

Preface i

Chapter 1: Reproductive Anatomy 1
    External Genitalia 1
    Vagina 2
    Uterus 3
    Key Takeaways 6
    Quiz 6

Chapter 2: Diagnosis of Pregnancy 9
    Physical and History Findings 9
    Laboratory Findings 9
    Ultrasonography 14
    Using Ultrasound and HCG Levels Together 15
    Key Takeaways 16
    Quiz 16

Chapter 3: Physiology of Pregnancy 19
    Cardiovascular Changes 19
    Hematological Changes 20
    Urinary Tract Changes 20
    Respiratory Changes 20
    Gastrointestinal and Hepatobiliary Changes 21
    Endocrine Changes 21
    Dermatological Changes 22
    Other Pregnancy-related Symptoms 22
    Key Takeaways 23
    Quiz 23

Chapter 4: Antepartum 26
    Pre-pregnancy Healthcare 26
    Prenatal Care 26
    Prenatal Visits 27
    Ultrasound 28
    Multiple Marker Screening 29

Chorionic Villus Sampling ... 29

Amniocentesis ... 29

Gestational Diabetes Screening ... 30

Things to Discuss ... 31

The Zika Virus ... 31

Key Takeaways ... 32

Quiz ... 32

Chapter 5: Intrapartum ... **35**

Monitoring the Mother in the First Stage of Labor ... 35

Monitoring the Fetus in the First Stage of Labor ... 37

Monitoring the Labor Progress ... 39

Examining the Vagina in Labor ... 40

Managing the Partogram ... 41

Second Stage of Labor ... 41

Dealing with Shoulder Dystocia ... 44

The Episiotomy ... 44

The Third Stage of Labor ... 44

Management of Postpartum Hemorrhage ... 45

Analgesia in Intrapartum Care ... 46

Key Takeaways ... 46

Quiz ... 47

Chapter 6: Postpartum ... **50**

Postpartum Care in the Hospital ... 50

Postpartum Care at Home ... 52

Postpartum Birth Control ... 53

Breastfeeding Issues ... 53

Postpartum Psychiatric Conditions ... 53

Treatment of Postpartum Psychiatric Disorders ... 55

Key Takeaways ... 56

Quiz ... 56

Chapter 7: Medical Conditions in Pregnancy ... **60**

Hypertension and Pregnancy ... 60

Treatment of Hypertension in Pregnancy ... 61

Preeclampsia 63
Diabetes and Pregnancy 64
Infectious Diseases and Pregnancy 65
Food Poisoning 66
Sexually Transmitted Diseases 66
Medications and Pregnancy 68
Key Takeaways 69
Quiz 69

Chapter 8: Obstetrical Complications 72
Amniotic Fluid Complications 72
Placental Abruption 73
Ectopic Pregnancy 74
Miscarriage or Fetal Loss 75
Placenta Previa 77
Preeclampsia and Eclampsia 79
Key Takeaways 81
Quiz 81

Chapter 9: Infections in Pregnancy 84
Group B Streptococcus 84
Urinary Tract Infections 85
Bacterial Vaginosis 85
Listeriosis 86
Syphilis 88
Chlamydia 89
Gonorrhea 90
Key Takeaways 91
Quiz 91

Chapter 10: Twin Gestation 94
Twin Basic Facts 94
Managing the Twin Gestation 95
Twin Complications 95
The First Trimester in a Twin Pregnancy 96
The Second Trimester in a Twin Pregnancy 96

    The Third Trimester in a Twin Pregnancy 96

    Risks in a Twin Pregnancy 97

    Key Takeaways 97

    Quiz 98

Chapter 11: Spontaneous Abortions and Fetal Death **101**

    Spontaneous Abortion 101

    Risk Factors and Etiology for a Spontaneous Abortion 102

    Treatment of Spontaneous Abortions 103

    Psychological Issues after a Spontaneous Abortion 104

    Management of Fetal Demise 104

    Diagnosis of Fetal Demise 106

    Key Takeaways 106

    Quiz 107

Chapter 12: Contraception and Sterilization **110**

    Intrauterine Contraception 110

    Hormonal Methods of Birth Control 111

    Emergency Contraception 112

    Barrier Methods 112

    Fertility Awareness Methods of Contraception 113

    Tubal Ligation 113

    Key Takeaways 114

    Quiz 115

Summary **118**

Course Test Questions **120**

Course Test Answers **138**

Preface

This course is a complete discussion of the practice of obstetrics and common issues obstetricians may encounter. While obstetrics is generally practiced by an obstetrician/gynecologist, many family practice physicians also engage in obstetrical practice. The course intends to cover issues related to normal obstetrical care as well as the management of obstetrical complications.

The first chapter of the course reviews the reproductive anatomy of adult females, including external anatomy including the vulva, the labia majora, and the clitoris. It also covers internal reproductive anatomy, including the ovaries, uterus, and cervix.

In the second chapter of the course, the diagnosis of pregnancy will be discussed. In a modern obstetrical practice, pregnancy is diagnosed with blood testing of beta human chorionic gonadotropin, or beta HCG, urine pregnancy tests, and ultrasonography. Even with accurate laboratory and imaging techniques, pregnancy can be successfully diagnosed with a thorough menstrual history and a gynecological examination.

The third chapter of the course is devoted to the physiological changes that occur in pregnancy. Pregnancy affects many body systems, including the cardiovascular system, the respiratory system, the gastrointestinal tract, the kidneys and ureters, the endocrine system, and the skin. Changes that occur during pregnancy don't often return to normal until several months after the delivery.

The fourth chapter of the course is a synopsis of the antepartum care involved in a normal pregnancy. Women tend to see their obstetrician early the first trimester and are followed at routine visits throughout the pregnancy.

An extensive discussion of intrapartum care is covered in the fifth chapter. Women in labor and their fetuses require close observation during the labor process to reduce the risk of intrapartum complications. This chapter particularly focuses on the monitoring process that happens regarding the wellbeing of the mother and unborn fetus.

The sixth chapter of the course covers the postpartum period. The postpartum period begins when the placenta is delivered and ends at an arbitrary six-week checkup, although the woman will continue to experience post-pregnancy changes for many months after giving birth. There can be psychological changes that take place as late as twelve months after giving birth.

The seventh chapter of the course covers common medical conditions that may affect the pregnant woman. Some pregnancies are high risk from the beginning because of a maternal health problem, such as hypertension or diabetes. Other pregnancies become complicated by the development of health problems unrelated to the reproductive system but may be exacerbated by pregnancy.

The eighth chapter of the course is devoted to covering the various obstetrical complications that can happen in both normal and high-risk pregnancies. Most pregnancies are normal and result in full term, healthy babies but others are complicated by external and internal factors.

Infections during pregnancy will also be discussed. Most of the infections that affect a pregnancy are directly related to the female reproductive system, such as gonorrhea and chlamydia; however, infections such as listeriosis and human immunodeficiency virus are not related with the reproductive system but can have serious consequences for the fetus or neonate.

The tenth chapter of the course is a brief discussion of twin pregnancies. Twin pregnancies happen often enough that most doctors who participate in obstetrical care will encounter many twin gestations in their practice.

The eleventh chapter of the course is a thorough discussion of spontaneous abortions and fetal demise. Spontaneous abortions are miscarriages that happen prior to the twentieth week of pregnancy, while a fetal demise is fetal death that occurs after the twentieth week of gestation.

The last chapter of this course discusses contraception in women as well as the sterilization process. Most women of reproductive age will need contraception if they are sexually active and don't desire to be pregnant. A woman who feels she is finished with the reproductive process may elect to have a tubal ligation.

Chapter 1: Reproductive Anatomy

There are several parts to the female reproductive tract, some of which are directly related to the external genitalia and the female sexual organs. Other aspects of the female anatomy are a part of the female reproductive system and involved in the act of reproduction.

External Genitalia

The most obvious part of the external female genitalia is the vulva, which is also referred to as the pudendum. This is the part of the female genitalia that is visible upon external inspection of the woman's genitals. The vulva is made up of the mons pubis, which contains the pubic hair and a fatty tissue layer. The labia minora and labia majora are the inner and outer lips, which are layers of tissue that surround either side of the vaginal opening. The hymen is a fold of tissue that covers the vaginal opening prior to a woman's first sexual experience. The clitoris is a female sex organ that is the primary source for female sexual pleasure.

Figure 1 describes the normal external genitalia of the female:

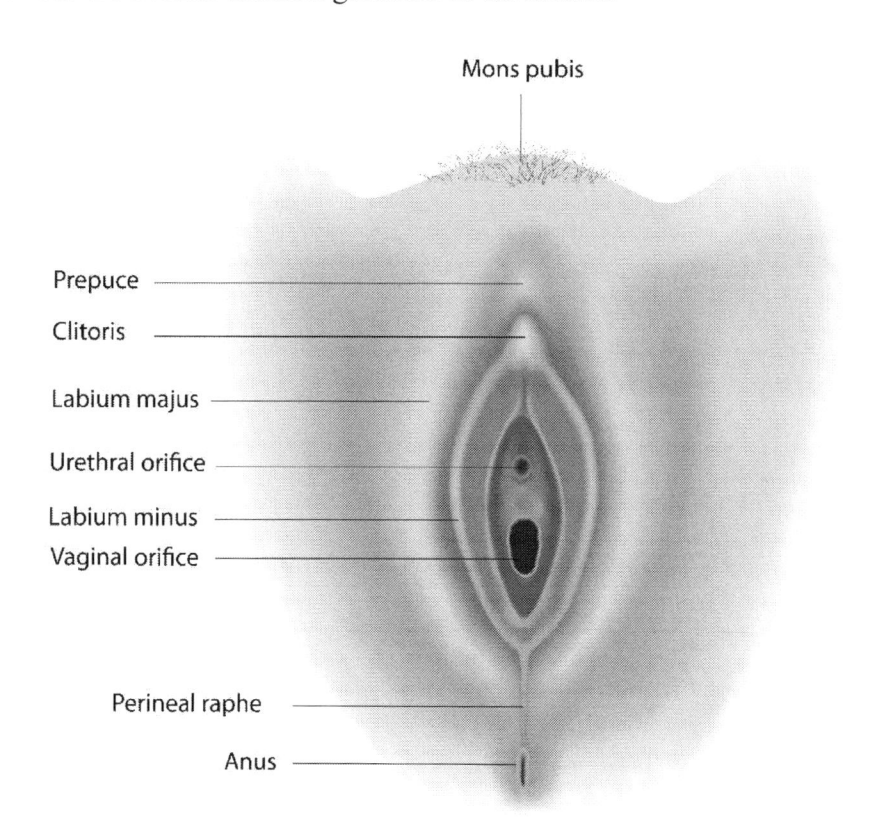

Figure 1

The primary anatomic boundaries that define the external genitalia include the mons pubis, which is on the anterior border of the external genitalia, the rectum, which forms the posterior border of the external genitalia, and the genitocrural folds or the thigh folds that make up the lateral margin of the genitalia.

The mons pubis can be identified as the round part of the vulva where the female pubic hair grows at the time of puberty. This area of the genitalia can be seen just anterior and superior to the pubic symphysis. The labia majora are the large tissue folds on either side of the vaginal opening. They consist mainly of fatty and fibrous tissue and contain hair follicles and a small amount of hair. The labia minora are the small folds, also referred to as nymphae. They are found just medial to the labia majora. They connect anteriorly to form the clitoris.

The hymen is a membrane covering the vaginal opening. It is usually not a complete membrane, having an opening that allows for the passage of menstrual tissue and menstrual blood. The clitoris is considered an erectile tissue, consisting of two crura, or folds, that are directly attached to the bony periosteum of the pubic bone. It is highly sensitive and the female equivalent to the male penile tissue.

Between the clitoris and the vaginal opening is the vestibule, which is a triangle-shaped area of tissue that contains the female urethra. The Skene glands open out into the vestibule as well as the Bartholin glands. The Skene glands and the Bartholin glands together lubricate the vaginal tissue. The vestibular bulbs are small areas of erectile tissue that are also situated in the tissues of the genitalia deep to the bulbocavernosus muscles.

Vagina

The vagina is the part of the female reproductive system that extends inward from the vulva, which is part of the female external genitalia, to the cervix, which marks the opening of the uterus. It resides wholly within the pelvis and can be found just anterior to the rectum. The anterior margin of the vagina is marked by the female urinary bladder. The uterus sits just above the vagina and can be found situated at a ninety-degree angle to the angle of the vaginal canal. The vagina is supported by pelvic ligaments and by connective tissue referred to as the endopelvic fascia.

Figure 2 describes the vagina and the rest of the female reproductive system:

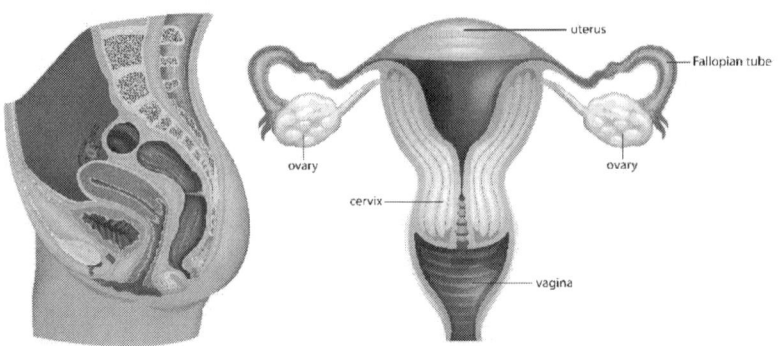

Figure 2

The lining tissues of the vagina include the rugae, which are folds along the length of the vagina. These can distend easily, allowing for penile insertion and the passage of the fetus during the act of childbearing. There are membranous tissues within the vagina, connective tissues, and erectile tissues. The main supportive structures of the vagina are the perineal membrane, the transverse peroneus muscles, and the urethral sphincter. There are perineal branches of the pudendal nerve that provide innervation to the vaginal tissues. The vagina is richly supplied by arteries, including a branch from the vaginal artery, which is a part of the internal iliac artery.

Most of the nerve supply to the vagina comes from the autonomic nervous system. There are sensory fibers extending from the sacral nerve roots that innervate the entire length of the vagina. There is adequate lymph drainage from the vagina that flows into the external iliac lymph nodes, the common and internal iliac lymph nodes, and the superficial inguinal lymph nodes.

Uterus

The uterus is an internal organ that is located in the midline of the pelvis, just between the female bladder and rectum. It is made from extremely thick and muscular walls and has an inner lining called the endometrium that responds to the changing hormonal state associated with the woman's monthly menstrual cycle.

There are two main parts of the uterus. The most inferior part of the uterus is the cervix, while the main part of the uterus is called the body or corpus uteri. Between the two parts of the uterus is the isthmus, which is a small area of constriction that separates them. The main body of the uterus is shaped like a globe and is situated at a ninety-degree angle to the angle of the vaginal canal.

The dome-shaped fundus is considered the most muscular aspect of the uterus, while the body of the uterus is the part of the female reproductive anatomy that contains the fetus, fluid, and placenta during pregnancy. During childbirth, the muscles of the uterus contract to expel the fetus.

The typical non-pregnant and nulliparous uterus weighs about forty to fifty grams. A uterus that isn't pregnant but has contained a previous pregnancy may weigh up to one hundred-ten grams. The uterus after menopause is atrophied and smaller than the uterus before menopause and will weigh less than forty grams.

The inside cavity of the uterus is flat and shaped like a triangle. The lateral tubes of the uterus extend out of the uterine cavity on either side of the uterus in the superolateral aspect of the structure. There are several ligaments and connective tissue structures that are supportive to the uterus.

The pelvic peritoneum is connected to the cervix and body of the uterus. It is called the broad ligament and reflects back upon the urinary bladder, extending to the sides of the uterus and connecting to the side walls of the pelvis on the lateral side walls. The cardinal ligament is another supportive structure composed of strands of connective tissue that also support the uterus.

There are rectouterine ligaments situated within the folds of the peritoneum, stretching from the posterior part of the cervix to connect to the sacrum. The round ligaments of the uterus are dense structures connecting the uterus to the anterolateral aspect of the abdominal wall. They are located inside the anterior folds of the broad ligament. The artery of Sampson is a small artery located within the round ligament that is ligated during a hysterectomy procedure. The rest of the blood supply to the uterus comes from the uterine arteries and the ovarian arteries.

There is a rich nerve supply and lymph drainage associated with the uterus. Lymph drainage from the uterus enters the lateral aortic lymph nodes, the pelvic lymph nodes, and the iliac lymph nodes—all of which surround the iliac blood vessels. The nerves supplying the uterus stem from the sympathetic nervous system and come from both the hypogastric nerve plexus and the ovarian nerve plexus. There is a parasympathetic aspect to the nerve supply to the uterus that stems from the pelvic splanchnic nerves derived from the second through fourth sacral nerves.

The cervix marks the lower aspect of the uterus and is the part of the uterus that separates the uterine body and the vaginal canal. The cervix is shaped like a cylinder and contains the endocervical canal that allows for the passage of seminal fluid into the uterus during sexual intercourse. It opens into the vagina by means of the external os, while the internal os represents the aspect of the uterus that opens during childbirth. The total length of the cervix is about three to five centimeters.

The main blood supply to the cervix stems from branches of the uterine artery, while the nerve supply comes from the uterine nerve. Most of the nerve supply to the cervix stems from the parasympathetic nervous system by means of the second through fourth sacral nerves. There are also pain fiber nerves that run along the parasympathetic nerves. There is a wide range of lymph nodes that drain from the cervix.

The uterine tubes or fallopian tubes are side appendages found on either side of the upper portion of the body of the uterus. They allow sperm to travel from the uterus to the egg, which has been released by the ovary at the time of ovulation. Once the egg is fertilized, it travels from the mid-portion of the fallopian tubes to the body of the uterus to be implanted. Each fallopian tube is about ten centimeters in length and about one centimeter in diameter.

Each is imbedded into a part of the uterine broad ligament known as the mesosalpinx. The most distal part of the fallopian tube widens out into fimbriae that encircle the ovary, allowing for a tighter connection between the fallopian tubes and the ovaries. The three main portions of the fallopian tubes are the isthmus, which is closest to the uterus, the ampulla, which is the middle portion of the tubes, and the distal infundibulum, which houses the fimbriae, which are necessary for catching the egg after ovulation.

The ovaries are connected loosely to the uterus by the fallopian tubes. There is one ovary on either side of the uterus. Each can be found inside the mesovarium part of the broad ligament. The ovaries are necessary for the hormonal component of the female reproductive system as well as to produce the female egg. Of the one to two million eggs inside the ovaries, only about three hundred are released as mature eggs that will be ripe enough for fertilization.

Figure 3 depicts the ovaries in relation to the uterus:

Diagram of Female Reproductive System

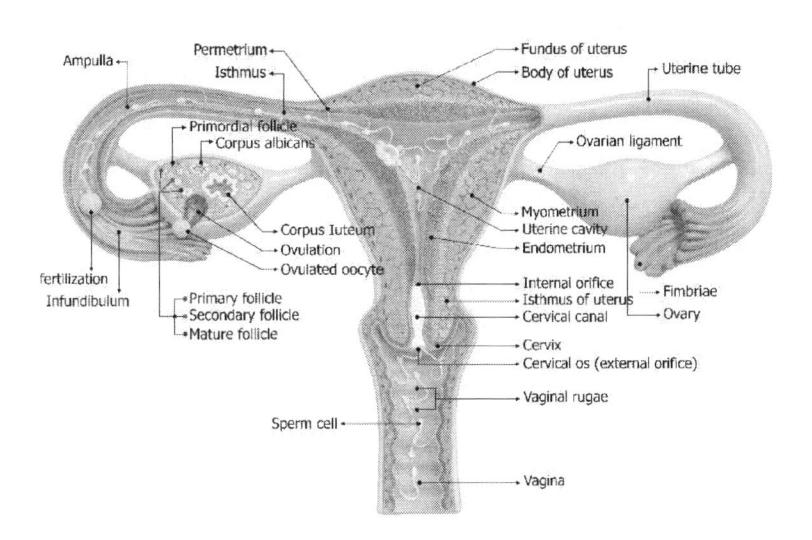

Figure 3

Each ovary is shaped like an oval and is gray in color. The surface of the ovaries is uneven and the ovarian size varies according to a woman's age and hormone status. The ovaries are as big as five centimeters in diameter during a woman's childbearing years, shrinking in size when a woman is into and past menopause. Cross-sectional cuts of the ovary will show multiple cysts of varied sizes, depending the stage of maturity of the ovarian follicle being represented.

There are several supporting ligaments to each ovary. The ovarian ligament is the piece of connective tissue that connects the uterus to the ovaries on either side of the ovary. The posterior aspect of the broad ligament gives rise to the mesovarium, which is a connective tissue layer that supports the ovarian structure and contains the blood supply to the ovaries. The infundibular pelvic ligament represents the suspensory ligament for the ovaries. There is a peritoneal fold covering the ovarian vessels that serves as an attachment for the ovary to the pelvic side walls.

The main blood supply to the ovaries comes from the ovarian arteries that extend from the ascending aorta, which branches off at about L2 of the vertebral column. The ovarian artery and the ovarian vein come out from the ovary at the hilum. The ovarian vein on the left drains into the left renal vein, while the ovarian vein on the right empties into the inferior vena cava. The nerve supply to the ovaries comes from the hypogastric plexus, the ovarian plexus, and the aortic plexus. There is lymph drainage to the ovaries that leads to the lateral aortic lymph nodes and the iliac lymph nodes.

Key Takeaways

- The female reproductive anatomy consists of the internal organs and the external genitalia.
- The main structure of the external genitalia in females is the vulva, which is the part of the female reproductive tract that lines either side of the vagina.
- The uterus is a large muscular structure that houses the fetus during pregnancy.
- The ovaries make up the hormonal aspect of the female reproductive system and make up the egg-releasing part of a woman's reproductive organs.

Quiz

1. Which part of the female reproductive anatomy is where the pubic hair originates?
    a. Mons pubis
    b. Labia minora
    c. Clitoris
    d. Labia majora

Answer: a. The mons pubis is the part of the female reproductive anatomy that is where the pubic hair originates.

2. You are evaluating the normal vaginal canal of an adult female. What part of the vagina allows for distention of the canal during childbirth?
    a. Suspensory ligaments
    b. Rugae
    c. Hymen
    d. Erectile tissues

Answer: b. The rugae are folds of connective tissue that stretch, allowing for distention of the vagina during childbirth.

3. Which part of the female reproductive anatomy is considered an erectile structure?
    a. Hymen
    b. Labia minora
    c. Clitoris
    d. Skene gland

Answer: c. The clitoris is the main erectile structure of the female reproductive anatomy and is responsible for the female sexual responsiveness.

4. Which part of the female reproductive anatomy is only an intact structure prior to the onset of menses?
    a. Clitoris
    b. Hymen
    c. Labia minora
    d. External os of the cervix

Answer: b. The hymen is a membranous structure that is generally only intact in childhood, breaking at the time of first intercourse or during some time prior to the onset of menses.

5. Which aspect of the female reproductive anatomy changes monthly as the woman's menstrual hormones change?
    a. Fallopian tubes
    b. Endometrium
    c. External cervical os
    d. Vaginal rugae

Answer: b. The character of the endometrium changes continuously and varies in character according to the hormonal changes associated with the menstrual cycle.

6. Roughly how many mature eggs are released from the female ovaries during childbearing years?
    a. Fifty
    b. One hundred
    c. Three hundred
    d. One thousand

Answer: c. About three hundred mature eggs are released from the female ovaries during a woman's childbearing years.

7. Which ligament is considered the suspensory ligament of the ovaries?
    a. Broad ligament
    b. Ovarian ligament
    c. Mesovarium
    d. Infundibular pelvic ligament

Answer: d. The infundibular pelvic ligament lies on either side of the uterus and is responsible for suspending the ovaries in the pelvis.

8. On histological evaluation of the ovaries, what main thing can be visualized?
    a. Sheets of immature egg cells in columns
    b. Connective tissue bands supporting immature egg cell structures
    c. Cystic structures of varying sizes representing follicles of different ages
    d. Scar tissue islands representing sclerosed follicles

Answer: c. Histological evaluation of the ovaries will reveal cystic structures of varying sizes, which represent follicles of different ages.

9. Which artery supplies the ovaries?
    a. Uterine artery
    b. Artery of Sampson
    c. Ovarian artery
    d. Iliac artery

Answer: c. The main arterial supply to the ovaries comes directly from the ovarian artery. There is one such artery located on each side of the uterus.

10. In evaluating the size and weight of the uterus, which woman would likely have the smallest uterine weight in grams?
    a. A pre-adolescent female
    b. A nulligravida 25-year-old female
    c. A multigravida 30-year-old female
    d. A 70-year-old postmenopausal female

Answer: d. Women past menopause have a highly-atrophied uterus that will weigh the least out of the choices given.

Chapter 2: Diagnosis of Pregnancy

Traditionally, history and physical examination findings determined the presence or absence of a pregnancy. In modern times, this is used along with diagnostic testing that can determine a woman's pregnancy status without an examination. Currently, both the physical evaluation and laboratory studies are used to identify the presence of a pregnancy.

Physical and History Findings

The usual diagnosis of pregnancy comes from the history of a woman's menstrual cycle and the findings on the physical examination. The main findings regarding the woman's history is the identification of the menstrual pattern of the newly pregnant woman. While diagnosing the pregnancy, the main history findings include the date of the last menstrual period, any abnormal periods, the use of contraceptives, and a history of any irregularity of the menstrual period. Up to a quarter of women have bleeding in the first trimester, which complicates the pregnancy assessment.

While assessing the pregnancy, the medical doctor must evaluate for findings suggestive of an ectopic pregnancy. These findings would include a rising human chorionic gonadotropin or HCG level along with an empty uterus on ultrasound, vaginal bleeding, and pain in the abdomen. Unfortunately, ectopic pregnancies are a major cause of death in the first trimester of pregnant women. For this reason, the diagnosis of ectopic pregnancy must be made prior to the rupture of the fallopian tubes.

Other things that might lead a doctor to the diagnosis of an ectopic pregnancy include the historical presence of a previous tubal pregnancy, the presence of or history of pelvic inflammatory disease, fallopian tube disease, or the use of an intrauterine device prior to the pregnancy. Previous tubal ligation or fertility therapies also predict the presence of an ectopic pregnancy. By history, there will be a suggestion of pregnancy symptoms and physical findings linked to a lack of a uterine pregnancy.

In the physical examination of a pregnant woman, the typical finding is that of an enlarged uterus, changes in the breast exam, and the softening of the cervix that is typically seen at about six weeks' gestation. This softening is referred to as a Hegar sign. The Chadwick sign can also be found, which is a bluish color of the cervix secondary to vascular congestion. A positive Chadwick sign can be found at around eight to ten weeks' gestation. The pregnant uterus can be palpated below the pelvic symphysis prior to twelve weeks' gestation and above the pelvic symphysis after twelve weeks' gestation. The gold standard for the identification of a healthy pregnancy on examination is the presence of a fetal heartbeat using a Doppler device or fetoscope.

Laboratory Findings

Several different hormones can be measured in a bloodwork evaluation of a pregnant woman that can help to diagnose a pregnancy. The most commonly used assay for pregnancy is the beta subunit of human chorionic gonadotropin or beta HCG level. There is also a test for the progesterone level and for a test known as the "early pregnancy factor". Both the cytotrophoblast and the syncytiotrophoblast secrete hormones in the pregnancy, including gonadotropin releasing hormone, corticotropin releasing hormone, somatostatin, human chorionic thyrotropin, inhibin, human placental lactogen, and several other hormones. While these hormones may be elevated in pregnancy, there is no testing available for the diagnosis of pregnancy.

The HCG molecule is a glycoprotein that is similar to follicle stimulating hormone, thyrotropin, and luteinizing hormone. The alpha subunit is closely connected to these hormones, while the beta subunit is different from the other hormones and has a thirty-amino acid tailpiece. The beta subunit core fragment is what is detected in the urine of pregnant women.

Histologically, the beta HCG subunit can be found in the syncytial layer of the blastomere in the embryo. Hyperglycosylated human chorionic gonadotropin is a type of HCG seen in the invasive cells of the embryo during implantation. Human chorionic gonadotropin messenger RNA can be found in blastomeres consisting of eight to ten cells at two days' gestation, but can't be isolated from a culture source until about six days. It can be found in maternal serum and maternal urine after about six days' post-implantation. This subunit of HCG may not be identified until after implantation has occurred and a vascular connection has been established allowing HCG to be transferred from the embryo to the blood of the woman.

HCG can be found in the maternal circulation as an intact dimer, as an alpha subunit, or as a beta subunit. The degraded form or core fragment is also found in the serum as well. The beta core fragment is the main form of HCG found after the fifth week of gestation. The intact and beta subunit of HCG have a great degree of day-to-day variability and are generally not detectable after ten days into the pregnancy. Ideally, the tests for the detection of pregnancy should be able to identify all types of the HCG molecule.

There are four main types of HCG assays. The first is the radioimmunoassay, immunoradiometric assay, fluoroimmunoassay, and the enzyme-linked immunosorbent assay or ELISA test. They are extremely specific for the HCG with antibodies available for binding to at least two isotopes of the intact HCG molecule. Most early pregnancy tests can detect pregnancy when the HCG molecule has a concentration of about twenty-five milli-International (mIU) Units per milliliter. Urine tests can identify the hyperglosylated HCG, which is the main form of the HCG substance used to detect a pregnancy.

Characteristic of the different assays include the following:

- The radioimmunoassay can detect HCG levels as low as five mIU per ml and takes about four hours to complete. It can be first felt to be positive at ten to eighteen days after conception or at about three to four weeks' gestation.
- The immunoradiometric assay is only sensitive when the HCG level is one hundred fifty mIU per ml and takes a half hour to complete. It is positive at eighteen to twenty-two days after conception or sometime after four weeks' gestation.
- Immunoradiometric assays have a poor sensitivity, detecting HCG levels at one thousand five hundred mIU/ml. It takes only two minutes to complete and is only detectable twenty-five to twenty-eight days after conception, or at five weeks' gestation.
- The Enzyme-Linked Immunosorbent Assay or ELISA takes eighty minutes to complete and can identify HCG levels as low as twenty-five mIU per milliliter.

- The fluoroimmunoassay is highly sensitive, able to detect a pregnancy at one mIU per milliliter. It takes two to three hours to perform and is positive fourteen to seventeen days after conception or at about three and a half weeks' gestation.

While HCG in its dimeric form as well as alpha and beta subunits are made within the pituitary gland of women who aren't pregnant and released into the bloodstream with luteinizing hormone, the levels are extremely low and cannot be detected with standard pregnancy testing.

In some cases, serial HCG levels are recommended. HCG can be detected in about five percent of patients after eight days' post-conception. This level rises to ninety-eight percent at the eleventh day post-conception. At four weeks' gestation, both the dimer and beta subunits double about every forty-eight hours. The doubling time at nine weeks' gestation is only about three and a half days. The levels peak at ten to twelve weeks' gestation, declining quickly after this until about twenty-two weeks' gestation, when there is a gradual rise until the time of the child's birth.

The initial rise is important in detecting the difference between a healthy and an unhealthy pregnancy, marred by being ectopic or by being a spontaneous abortion. Women whose HCG levels do not double at the appropriate time should be evaluated an abnormal pregnancy. The clinical picture must be considered as well as the laboratory values found. Ectopic pregnancies and spontaneous abortions often have a low rise in HCG level that can be identified with serial HCG levels. However, normal rises in HCG levels do not exclude the presence of an ectopic pregnancy.

When the medical doctor encounters elevated levels of beta HCG or a rapid rise the levels, this can mean the pregnancy is abnormal, such as is found in a molar pregnancy, fetal chromosomal abnormalities, or multiple gestation pregnancies.

False positive HCG levels can be found in certain medical conditions, but these are extremely rare, with an incidence rate of less than two percent. Falsely positive HCG levels arise from non-HCG substances that interfere with the HCG testing or by the detection of HCG that is made by the pituitary gland. Human luteinizing hormone levels can interfere as can rheumatoid factor, anti-animal immunoglobulin antibodies, binding proteins, and heterophile antibodies. The serum levels detected are generally less than one thousand mIU per milliliter and can be detected as low as one hundred fifty mIU per milliliter. There are several methods available to help identify a false positive HCG test. A urine test can be done after a blood test, which will confirm a real pregnancy. False positive rates are rare during a urine test as the molecules that interfere with the test are too big to be excreted in the urine.

There are other ways to verify the presence of a false positive HCG level. The medical doctor can retest the same specimen, test a different specimen, or do serial measurements, evaluating for a specified risk in the HCG level over time. The major sources of a positive HCG test other than pregnancy include the following:

- There can be a phantom HCG test, in which heterophile antibodies bind together, causing an antibody reaction despite the absence of an antigen. Antibody formation is secondary to exposure to animals used to make the assay antibodies. The best way to handle this is to do a urine HCG level.
- There can be pituitary HCG that is stimulated by the hypothalamic release of gonadotropin releasing hormone and blocked by gonadotropin releasing hormone antagonist agents and

estrogen/progesterone therapy. This may occur in postmenopausal women who have elevated levels of gonadotropin releasing hormone. This can be further identified by giving the woman birth control pills, which decreases the HCG levels.
- The patient may have exogenous intake of HCG. This is used by some centers to help in weight loss by giving HCG orally or intramuscularly. Repeat HCG assays might be negative if exogenous administration is discontinued for at least twenty-four hours.
- There can be a trophoblastic cancer, which is made up from placental fragments, a trophoblastic cancer, or placental site trophoblastic cancer.
- There can be a gestational trophoblastic cancer involves a consistent low-level amount of human chorionic gonadotropin without any evidence of primary or metastatic cancer. Frequent HCG levels should be measured, and if a rise occurs, active gestational trophoblastic neoplasia should be considered.
- There can be placental site trophoblastic cancer that can be identified as having low levels of HCG along with intramyometrial lesions identified on ultrasound.
- There can be a non-trophoblastic cancer that can be secreted from a variety of reproductive and nonreproductive cancers. These include stomach cancer, pancreatic cancer, liver cancer, lung cancer, uterine cancer, bladder cancer, or testicular cancer.

Urine testing for HCG may produce a false negative, secondary to urine that is too diluted or HCG levels that are too low. The main reasons for a negative test is that the HCG level in the urine is too low to be detected by ordinary urine testing. The test may be too low because the woman miscalculated the date of her missed menstrual period or had a delayed menses from an early pregnancy loss. Delayed ovulation or delayed implantation can also result in low HCG concentrations at the time of testing.

Progesterone levels can be helpful in identifying an abnormal early pregnancy. Serum progesterone reflects progesterone production by the corpus luteum, which is highly active in cases of a normal pregnancy. The measurement of serum progesterone levels is cheap and extremely reliable in predicting the prognosis of a given pregnancy. As of now, radio-immunoassays and fluoro-immunoassays are available that can be performed in under four hours. A dipstick ELISA test that can determine a serum progesterone of less than fifteen nanograms per milliliter is available for medical doctors to use in pregnancy testing. It can be used for populations at risk as progesterone levels of higher than fifteen nanograms per milliliter make it nearly impossible that an ectopic pregnancy is present.

A viable intrauterine gestation can be identified with more than ninety-seven percent sensitivity if the serum progesterone levels are higher than twenty-five nanograms per milliliter. On the other hand, serum progesterone levels of less than five nanograms per milliliter can identify a nonviable gestation with about a hundred percent accuracy. However, it does not indicate the difference between an ectopic pregnancy and a spontaneous abortion. If the progesterone level is between these low and high values, more testing is necessary to establish the health of the pregnancy through other means.

Early pregnancy factor, or EPF, may be more useful to detect pregnancies in the future. It is an undefined immunosuppressive protein that shows up shortly after conception and is quicker to detect than an HCG level. It is almost undetectable at the time of a fetus's birth. It is elevated within forty-eight hours after a successful in vitro fertilization. It cannot be detected within twenty-four hours after childbirth or after treatment for an ectopic or intrauterine pregnancy. EPF is not detected in spontaneous abortions or ectopic pregnancies so when absent, it may portend a bad outcome to the pregnancy.

EPF cannot be used to diagnose a pregnancy at this time because it is difficult to isolate. It relies on a complicated test process called the rosette inhibition test. It may be a more prominent test in the diagnosis of conception before implantation as it is highly accurate in the dating process in future pregnancies once the technology becomes available.

Most pregnancies are identified with home pregnancy tests. These tests employ the modern immunometric assay and claim a ninety-nine percent accuracy. The truth is they are only accurate at ninety-nine percent if the test is taken on the day of the missed period, even though some women will have a positive test up to four to five days before a missed period. This means if a woman tests herself before the day of the missed period, the accuracy is much less than ninety-nine percent, making the claims of these types of tests somewhat misleading.

Figure 4 shows a typical home pregnancy test:

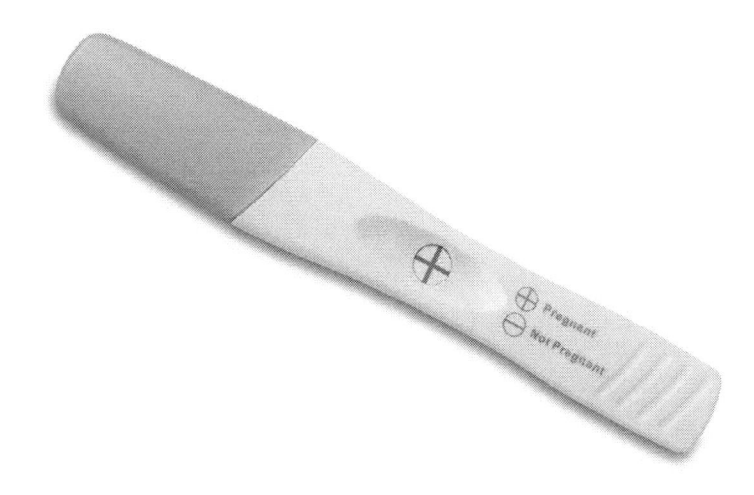

Figure 4

Most home pregnancy tests are used during the fourth completed gestational week. Urine HCG values are extremely variable during this period and can be as little as twelve mIU per milliliter or as high as two thousand five hundred mIU per milliliter. This extreme variability in HCG levels persists into the fifth gestational week, when the values can be as low as thirteen mIU per ml or as high as six thousand mIU per milliliter. This means that home pregnancy tests that can detect HCG levels as low as twenty-five percent have a chance of being falsely negative. A hundred percent accuracy can only be achieved when the HCG level is a hundred mIU per milliliter, which may not occur until after the missed period. Digital tests tend to be more accurate and easier to interpret than other tests.

Serum HCG levels are used in the diagnosis of an early successful pregnancy in women who have undergone in vitro fertilization and embryo transfer. Serum HCG levels two weeks after an embryo transfer portend a good pregnancy outcome. Quantitative HCG levels are interpreted as follows: If the level is less than three hundred mIU per milliliter, the success of the pregnancy is only nine percent; If the level is between three hundred and six hundred mIU per milliliter, the success of the pregnancy is about fifty percent, while an HCG level in the serum of higher than six hundred mIU per milliliter, indicates a successful pregnancy at about a hundred percent.

Ultrasonography

Transvaginal ultrasonography or TVUS allows for the diagnosis of a healthy pregnancy much earlier than the standard transabdominal ultrasound or TAUS. Ultrasound is also invaluable in following uncomplicated pregnancies for dating purposes and can screen a pregnancy for obvious fetal physical anomalies. It isn't used to diagnose a pregnancy unless there is evidence of vaginal bleeding or abdominal pain during the first trimester or when the patient's pregnancy is high risk. TVUS is extremely accurate in confirming an intrauterine pregnancy and can be used to accurately determine the patient's obstetrical dates when used early in the first trimester of pregnancy.

There are many reasons to employ TVUS as opposed to TAUS during the pregnancy. TVUS can show a viable intrauterine pregnancy a week sooner than can be identified with TAUS. Patients don't have to have a full bladder nor need they suffer the discomfort of pressing on the lower abdomen with a full bladder. Obese women can be much better evaluated with TVUS as opposed to the TAUS procedure. The major downside of doing a TVUS is some women experience discomfort from the vaginal probe.

Figure 5 shows what a transvaginal ultrasound probe looks like:

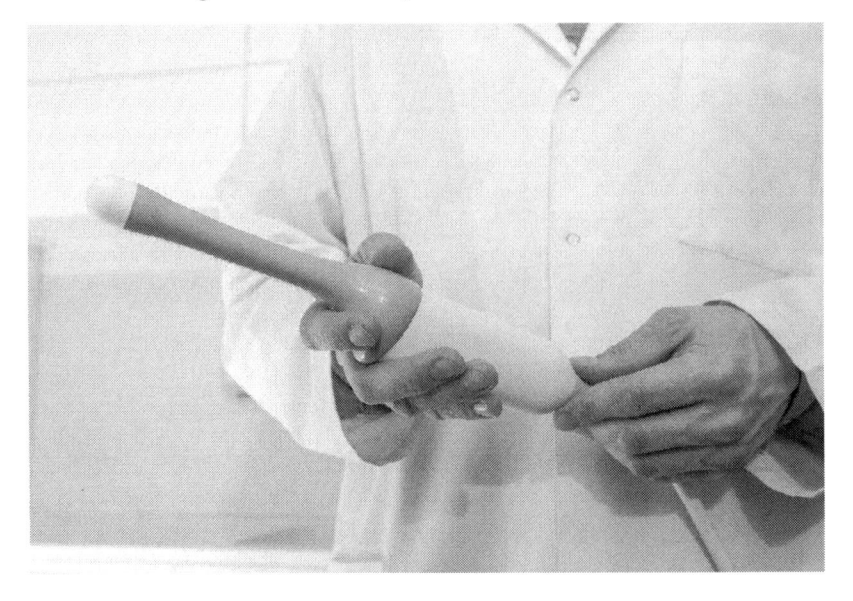

Figure 5

There is a higher frequency of ultrasound testing with TVUS when compared to TAUS. The TVUS uses frequencies in the range of five to ten megahertz, while the TAUS employs frequencies in the range of three to five megahertz. The higher frequency in TVUS allows for better resolution of the image but is less able to penetrate tissues, thus the need for a transvaginal insertion. The first thing identified during this exam is the gestational sac, which can be identified by four to five weeks gestation. It grows about a millimeter per day. By six weeks gestation, the ultrasound can identify a double decidual sign, which involves the finding of an area of thickened decidua around the gestational sac. Because the presence of a gestational sac can be confused with a fluid or blood-filled cyst in the uterus, the diagnosis of a healthy pregnancy can only be made after viewing the surrounding decidua.

On the other hand, the yolk sac, which is a small circular structure on ultrasound with a fluid-filled center, can be seen by about four to five weeks gestation, which can portend the presence of a healthy pregnancy. The yolk sac is usually seen prior to the finding of a gestational sac being larger than ten centimeters. This means that, if the yolk sack is bigger than seven centimeters and there is no evidence of a fetal pole on examination, the likelihood of an abnormal pregnancy is high. A gestational sac bigger than ten millimeters in the absence of a yolk sac is extremely rare. This finding would most likely indicate an unhealthy pregnancy or inevitable spontaneous abortion. The technical term for this is a blighted ovum or an anembryonic pregnancy.

Yolk sacs bigger than seven millimeters without a fetal pole identify a nonviable pregnancy and will be helpful in excluding an ectopic pregnancy because it identifies the gestational tissues as being intrauterine, even though the pregnancy is not healthy. Unfortunately, there is a one out of three thousand chance of having both an intrauterine pregnancy and an ectopic pregnancy, so the presence of an intrauterine yolk sac does not completely rule out an ectopic pregnancy.

A fetal pole or embryonic pole can be seen at five to six weeks gestational age. It should be evaluated using a TVUS procedure because it can only be identified when the gestational sac is about eighteen millimeters in diameter. In contrast, TAUS requires the gestational sac to be bigger than two and a half centimeters before the fetal pole can be identified. The fetal pole is a solid structure on ultrasound that grows about one millimeter per day after it first visualized.

Motion of the heart may be seen when the embryo is only two to three millimeters in diameter but is virtually always detected when the embryo is about five millimeters in diameter. At about five to six weeks' gestation, the heart rate will be about a hundred to one hundred fifteen beats per minute but will increase steadily to an average of about a hundred and forty beats per minute by the ninth week of gestation.

Using Ultrasound and HCG Levels Together

The ultrasound is most helpful when it is used in conjunction with HCG level testing. The findings seen on a transvaginal ultrasound closely correlate with specific quantitative HCG levels. This is referred to as a discriminatory level. This is the level of HCG at which a certain structure in question needs to be identified in the ultrasound evaluation of a normal and healthy singleton pregnancy located inside the uterus.

The gestational sac has been seen in a TVUS examination with an HCG level as low as three hundred mIU per milliliter, but it may take an HCG level of up to a thousand mIU per milliliter to be certain that the gestational sac can be identified. The discriminatory level for the finding of a gestational sac is about three thousand six hundred mIU per milliliter. If it isn't seen at this serum level, the medical doctor must look for other pathology. Some doctors use a discriminatory level of two thousand mIU per milliliter for the location of a gestational sac by means of TVUS and will look for pathology if the gestational sac isn't identified when the serum HCG level is at least two thousand mIU per ml. When using TAUS, the discriminatory value of HCG must be at least three thousand six hundred mIU per milliliters.

Even when an intrauterine pregnancy has been identified, the adnexa need to be evaluated to make sure there isn't an ectopic pregnancy. While the discriminatory level for the finding of a gestational sac using the TAUS procedure is only three thousand six hundred mIU per milliliter, the usual HCG level seen at this point in the pregnancy is generally greater than six thousand five hundred mIU per milliliter.

The usefulness of the transvaginal ultrasound in cases of a serum HCG level less than a thousand mIU per milliliter is controversial. Only about thirteen percent of unhealthy uterine pregnancies and thirty-nine percent of ectopic pregnancies can be detected by TVUS with HCG levels around a thousand mIU per milliliter. Even so, when the level is found to be this low, a transvaginal ultrasound should be performed to ensure there isn't an ectopic pregnancy or an inevitable spontaneous abortion.

The other structures seen at specific HCG levels are the yolk sac and the fetal pole. The yolk sac is usually seen with HCG levels of about two thousand five hundred mIU per milliliter, while the embryonic pole can usually be seen with HCG levels of at least five thousand. The fetal heartbeat can be identified in a normal pregnancy at HCG levels of about ten thousand mIU per liter. Because each pregnancy is different, these HCG levels are not absolute.

Key Takeaways

- Traditionally, a woman's menstrual history and a physical evaluation of the pelvic structures has been used to identify the presence of a pregnancy.
- The gold standard for the detection of a healthy pregnancy is the finding of a fetal heartbeat on a Doppler evaluation or by means of a fetoscope.
- HCG evaluations can be either urine qualitative tests or serum quantitative tests. There are many quantitative tests available, but these are not all used in clinical practice.
- The serum progesterone level and serum early pregnancy factor are other ways to diagnose a healthy pregnancy, but these are not currently in everyday use.
- A transvaginal ultrasound is preferable over a transabdominal ultrasound because it can detect the presence of a healthy pregnancy a week or so earlier than the TAUS procedure.
- The ultrasound can be used along with HCG testing to best evaluate the presence of a healthy pregnancy and to exclude an ectopic pregnancy or inevitable spontaneous abortion.

Quiz

1. You are evaluating a woman suspected of being pregnant. You palpate the uterus below the pubic symphysis. What can you determine on this basis?
   a. The woman has an ectopic pregnancy.
   b. The woman is in her second trimester of pregnancy.
   c. The woman is less than twelve weeks' gestation.
   d. The woman probably has an inevitable spontaneous abortion.

Answer: c. The finding of a uterine fundus that does not rise past the pubic symphysis means the pregnancy is less than twelve weeks' gestation. Even so, the possibility of an ectopic pregnancy or spontaneous abortion cannot be ruled in or out.

2. In evaluating a woman who you suspect to be pregnant, you notice a positive Chadwick sign. What is this from?
    a. Venous congestion of the cervix
    b. Thinning of the cervix
    c. The presence of endometrial cells at the external os of the cervix
    d. The presence of a cervix much lower in the vaginal canal than is seen in non-pregnant females

Answer: a. A positive Chadwick sign is a bluish discoloration of the cervix caused by venous congestion in the cervix. It can be seen on a vaginal speculum examination.

3. You are evaluating the pregnancy status of a 24-year-old female and note a specifically positive Hegar sign. What gestational age is likely to show this finding for the first time?
    a. Four weeks' gestation
    b. Six weeks' gestation
    c. Eight weeks' gestation
    d. Twelve weeks' gestation

Answer: b. A positive Hegar sign or softening of the uterus can easily be identified at about six weeks' gestation and beyond.

4. You are evaluating a woman who has a serum HCG level of three hundred mIU per milliliter but you suspect this might be a false positive as the patient's clinical presentation does not support a pregnancy. What lab testing can be done to show this?
    a. A serum progesterone level
    b. A serum early pregnancy factor level
    c. A urine qualitative pregnancy test
    d. A repeat serum HCG level in two days

Answer: c. If you suspect the serum HCG level is from a non-pregnancy source, there is no reason to repeat the test and the testing of progesterone and early pregnancy factor will not help. A urine test is almost exclusively found in pregnancy and can tell the difference between a pregnancy-related HCG elevation and a non-pregnancy-related HCG level.

5. You are trying to determine the health of a pregnancy by doing a transvaginal ultrasound to detect a fetal heartbeat. What fetal pole size should yield the finding of a heartbeat?
    a. Two millimeters
    b. Five millimeters
    c. 50 millimeters
    d. One centimeter

Answer: b. The fetal pole can be first identified by about five millimeters in diameter but, in unusual circumstances, it can be detected before this size.

6. You are attempting to determine the presence of a viable pregnancy early in the first trimester. At what progesterone level can you determine the presence of a healthy pregnancy to a reasonable degree of accuracy?
    a. Five nanograms per milliliter

b. Twenty-five nanograms per milliliter
c. Fifty nanograms per milliliter
d. Seventy-five nanograms per milliliter

Answer: d. The finding of a serum progesterone level of at least seventy-five nanograms per milliliter is indicative of a healthy intrauterine pregnancy.

7. You are doing a transvaginal ultrasound for a woman suspected of being newly pregnant. At what gestational age would you suspect to find the presence of a fetal pole?
    a. Four to five weeks
    b. Five to six weeks
    c. Six to seven weeks
    d. Seven to eight weeks

Answer: b. A fetal pole can be easily identified using a transvaginal ultrasound at about five to six weeks' gestational age.

8. Why should it be necessary to use transvaginal ultrasound along with HCG testing to identify a healthy pregnancy?
    a. Transvaginal ultrasounds are not very precise in identifying pregnancies before six weeks' gestation.
    b. The HCG level is better able to predict a healthy pregnancy when the ultrasound findings support the lab test.
    c. There are discriminatory levels that mean certain structures need to be present in a healthy pregnancy at certain HCG levels.
    d. The HCG alone cannot predict a healthy pregnancy.

Answer: c. Ultrasound and HCG testing can be helpful because there are certain discriminatory levels indicating when certain fetal structures can be seen at specific HCG levels.

9. There are many home pregnancy HCG tests. What type of testing is involved in these tests?
    a. Immunometric assay
    b. Immunoradiometric assay
    c. Enzyme-linked immunosorbent assay
    d. Radiometric assay

Answer: a. The basic urine home pregnancy test involves the use of an immunometric assay, which isn't very sensitive but can be done to avoid the false positive HCG levels that can be seen in serum testing.

10. You are evaluating a woman at about six weeks' gestational age by ultrasound. What is the importance of seeing a decidua?
    a. The presence of a decidua rules out an ectopic pregnancy.
    b. The presence of a decidua confirms a healthy intrauterine pregnancy.
    c. The presence of a decidua at six weeks' gestation means that the dates are inaccurate.
    d. The finding of a decidua doesn't necessarily identify an intrauterine pregnancy.

Answer: b. The finding of a decidua at six weeks' gestation generally confirms the presence of an intrauterine pregnancy. However, It does not rule out an ectopic pregnancy.

Chapter 3: Physiology of Pregnancy

The physiology of a pregnant woman involves bodily changes that are not necessarily directly related to the female reproductive tract rather bodily manifestations that occur because of a secondary tissue response to the hormonal changes during pregnancy. It should be noted that pregnancy lasts about two hundred sixty-six days after conception or about two hundred eighty days from the beginning of the last menstrual period prior to getting pregnant.

Cardiovascular Changes

When a woman is pregnant, the cardiac output increases by between thirty percent and fifty percent starting at about six weeks' gestation and reaching a peak output at about sixteen to twenty-eight weeks' gestation. The cardiac output is extremely sensitive to the woman's body position. As the woman becomes increasingly pregnant, the gravid uterus places pressure on the pelvic and abdominal vena cava, resulting in a decrease in cardiac output when lying flat. After thirty weeks' gestation, the cardiac output goes down but increases again during labor. After the birth of the infant, the uterus contracts sharply, decreasing the cardiac output so that it is only about fifteen to twenty-five percent above normal. It returns to normal by the sixth week following the birth.

The increase in cardiac output in a pregnant woman is due primarily to the high demands of the uteroplacental blood flow. The volume of blood necessary for adequate circulation of the uterus and placenta increase markedly, with circulation in the intervillous state acting as an arteriovenous shunt, which necessitates an increase in cardiac output.

To cause an increase in cardiac output, the heart rate will go up from about seventy beats per minute to about ninety beats per minute. The stroke volume increases as well. During the second trimester of pregnancy, the blood pressure generally drops, and the pulse pressure becomes wider in the absence of any change in angiotensin and renin levels. The reason for the widening of the pulse pressure is the presence of the placental intervillous space and a decreased vascular resistance. During the third trimester, however, the blood pressure becomes normal again. Twin pregnancies have a lower blood pressure overall when compared to the singleton pregnancy. The oxygen consumption goes up in pregnancy as well.

This hyperdynamic circulatory state in pregnancy will mean a higher frequency of benign functional heart murmurs and the accentuation of the heart sounds. An x-ray or electrocardiogram of the heart in pregnancy will show displacement of the heart to the left and a slight left-sided rotation. It is common to have benign premature atrial contractions and premature ventricular contractions in pregnancy that necessitate only reassurance. The finding of paroxysmal atrial tachycardia is also significantly found in pregnancy and may necessitate the use of prophylactic antiarrhythmic medications or digitalis. Even cardioversion can be used in pregnancy as this does not adversely affect the fetus.

Hematological Changes

The total blood volume in pregnancy goes up, but there is a disproportionate increase in plasma with about a one thousand six hundred milliliter gain in plasma volume or about a fifty percent increase. By contrast, the RBC mass only increases by twenty-five percent, resulting in the presence of a dilutional anemia. This effect is more profound in twin pregnancies, which causes an increase in blood volume that can be as high as sixty percent. The white blood cell count also increases in pregnancy and it is not unusual to see WBC counts between nine thousand and twelve thousand cells per microliter. Extreme leukocytosis of greater than twenty thousand cells per microliter can be seen during labor the days following the birth.

The iron requirements of a pregnant woman go up, so the total iron intake recommended in pregnancy is increased by about one gram throughout the whole pregnancy. Women in the last half of pregnancy need about six to seven milligrams of elemental iron per day. The placenta and fetus take about three hundred milligrams of iron during the pregnancy, while the increased red blood cell mass takes about five hundred milligrams. About two hundred grams of iron are excreted by the body. This means that a pregnant woman needs increased iron intake through the diet and supplementation. Iron supplements are needed because a woman's iron stores, which are only about three hundred to five hundred milligrams, and dietary intake does not often meet the iron requirements of pregnancy.

Urinary Tract Changes

There are changes in the kidney function of a pregnant woman that go along with an increase in cardiac output. The renal glomerular filtration rate increases by about thirty to fifty percent during pregnancy, peaking between sixteen and twenty-four weeks' gestation, maintaining an elevated level until the birth of the child. The blood urea nitrogen or BUN level goes down to less than ten milligrams per deciliter and the serum creatinine level decreases in proportion to this, with levels of about 0.5 to 0.7 milligrams per deciliter. A significant degree of distention of the ureters can be found, which is called a hydroureter. This caused by the ureter's response to elevated progesterone levels in pregnancy and by the direct effect of pressure being placed on the ureters from the expanding uterus. It may take up to twelve weeks' postpartum to resolve the hydroureter.

Postural changes can affect the kidney function more during the pregnancy than at other times in a woman's life. The supine position increases the kidney function to a greater degree, while standing up decreases the kidney function. Kidney function is greatly increased in the lateral position, especially when the woman lies on her left side. When lying on the left side, the pressure causes a secondary increase in kidney function. This recumbent change in kidney function accounts for the fact that pregnant women need to urinate more often during the night.

Respiratory Changes

There are respiratory changes that will generally occur during pregnancy secondary to the reactivity of the lungs to progesterone elevations. The presence of progesterone causes a lowering of carbon dioxide levels in the blood. To accomplish this, the tidal volume of respiration and the respiratory rate will increase. This causes an increase in the blood pH level. Oxygen consumption increases by about twenty percent in pregnancy to meet the demands of the maternal organs, the fetus itself, and the placenta. There is also a decrease in the inspiratory and expiratory reserve, residual lung volume, blood CO2 level, and lung capacity. The blood oxygen level and the vital capacity don't change. Surprisingly, there is an increase in the woman's thoracic circumference by about ten centimeters.

An evaluation of the respiratory tract will reveal a great deal of hyperemia and edema of the tissues of the lungs. There can be hyperemia and swelling of the nasal passages as well as nasopharyngeal obstruction from the hormonal influences of the pregnancy. The Eustachian tubes can be blocked on a temporary basis. The woman's voice may change in quality and tone during pregnancy. It is also more common to have shortness of breath while exercising during pregnancy as well as the finding of deeper respirations.

Gastrointestinal and Hepatobiliary Changes

As a pregnancy continues, there will be pressure on the stomach from the expanding uterus as well as pressure on the colon and rectum, leading to constipation. There is a necessary decrease in gastrointestinal motility, which is largely secondary to serum progesterone level increases that cause a relaxation of gastrointestinal smooth muscle. It is extremely common to have heartburn and an increase in belching from a relaxation in the lower esophageal sphincter and delayed gastric emptying. The presence of a hiatal hernia in the woman will only increase heartburn symptoms. There is a relative decrease in the stomach's secretion of hydrochloric acid. This basically means that peptic ulcer disease is not very common in pregnant woman. Even women with pre-pregnancy gastric ulcers will have partial resolution of their symptoms.

Whether there is an increase in gallbladder problems in pregnancy is controversial. There appears to be minor changes in a woman's liver function in pregnancy and, the bile transportation abilities. The liver enzymes will be normal except for the alkaline phosphatase level, which increases in the third trimester of pregnancy, peaking at term when the level can be up to three times the normal level. This increase is not due to maternal alkaline phosphatase production but comes from the placenta.

Endocrine Changes

Pregnancy changes the functionality of most of a woman's endocrine gland, in part because the placenta makes its own hormones. In addition, most hormones made by the body are circulating along with bloodborne proteins, and there are more proteins during pregnancy.

The placenta is responsible for making the beta subunit of HCG, which is a trophic hormone that, like FSH and LH, helps to maintain the corpus luteum, preventing any further ovulations that might take place. The levels of estrogen and progesterone increase, in part because of ongoing stimulation by beta HCG, which stimulates ovarian production of these hormones. After about the ninth or tenth weeks' gestation, the placenta is capable making its own estrogen and progesterone to help maintain the pregnancy.

The placenta produces another hormone that is chemically like thyroid stimulating hormone. This stimulates the female thyroid gland, resulting in thyroid tissue hyperplasia, increased blood vessel supply to the thyroid gland, and thyroid enlargement. Estrogen also causes a stimulation of the liver cells, which in turn make more thyroid binding globulin. Thus, while there is an elevation in bound thyroxine and triiodothyronine in the maternal circulation, the free levels of these hormones are completely normal. However, the clinical picture may mimic that of hyperthyroidism with symptoms such as excessive perspiration, palpitations, tachycardia, and emotional difficulties. The actual incidence of true hyperthyroidism in pregnant women is only about 0.08 percent.

The placenta also produces corticotropic hormone or CRH, which causes a stimulation of the ACTH hormone secretion by the pituitary gland. This causes a secondary rise in adrenal hormones cortisol and aldosterone. This can cause peripheral edema. Increased production of corticosteroids and placental progesterone results in an increased resistance to insulin and an increased bodily requirement for insulin. The elevated levels of human placental lactogen and the increase in the stress of pregnancy also contribute to insulin resistance. The placenta also makes insulinase, which breaks down insulin, thereby increasing the maternal requirements for insulin. This what leads to the development of gestational diabetes or frank diabetes. The placenta also makes melanocyte-stimulating hormone or MSH, which increases the skin pigmentation in the latter half of the pregnancy.

The pituitary gland gets bigger by about one hundred thirty-five percent in pregnancy. The maternal plasma prolactin level increases by a factor of ten. Increased serum prolactin levels contribute to thyrotropin releasing hormone increases. The main function of prolactin elevations in the pregnant female is to stimulate lactation. The level becomes normal after childbirth, even in situations where the woman breastfeeds her infant.

Dermatological Changes

Increased levels of estrogen, progesterone, and melanocyte stimulating hormone cause pigment changes to occur in the woman's skin. The exact mechanism of action of this is unknown but one can find many pregnant women with melasma or "mask of pregnancy", which is a darkening of the skin of the cheeks and forehead in pregnant women. The areola, axilla, and genitalia are darkened, and many women have a linea nigra, which is a dark line appearing from the umbilicus to the pubic symphysis. The pigment changes often take a year to dissipate. Spider angiomata and visible varicose veins in the legs are extremely common because of excess pressure on the venous system by the expanding uterus.

Other Pregnancy-related Symptoms

Because of the elevation in estrogen and progesterone in pregnancy, the woman will experience breast engorgement, which are similar to changes seen in premenstrual syndrome but can be even more prominent. Nausea and vomiting care common because of high estrogen levels and high human chorionic gonadotropin levels. These begin to rise within ten days after conception. The corpus luteum produces large amounts of estrogen and progesterone under the influence of placental HCG production. A side effect of these hormones is often fatigue and abdominal bloating.

A pelvic examination will reveal the presence of a softer cervix and a soft, larger uterus. The cervix is bluish in color from venous congestion in the pelvic area. At about twelve weeks' gestation, the uterus can be palpated on examination of the abdomen as it has finally risen above the level of the pubic symphysis. At twenty weeks' gestation, the uterine fundus rises to the level of the umbilicus, while at term, it reaches up to the level of the female xyphoid process located at the superior margin of the abdomen.

Generally, the urine and blood tests are used to diagnose a pregnancy and the tests will be relatively accurate, even when the woman has yet to miss her period. Normally, the qualitative HCG test is enough to confirm a pregnancy; however, serial quantitative serum HCGs can be done a couple of days apart to tell the difference between a healthy and unhealthy pregnancy. The acceptable doubling of the quantitative HCG level is about two days in pregnancies under two months' gestation.

Other reproductive changes that can be present in pregnancy and can be used to diagnose the pregnancy include finding a gestational sac at four to five weeks on ultrasound along with an HCG level of at least one thousand five hundred mIU per milliliter. Yolk sacs can be seen at five weeks' gestation. Fetal heartbeats can be seen on ultrasound at five to six weeks, while Doppler ultrasonography can confirm a pregnancy around eight to ten weeks. Fetal movements can be felt by the mother and by her doctor after the twentieth week of gestation.

Key Takeaways

- There are numerous changes in the maternal body because of pregnancy hormones that don't directly relate to the female reproductive tract.
- Pregnancy is a hypermetabolic state because the placenta and fetus contribute to the state of metabolism in the pregnant woman.
- The main gastrointestinal symptoms seen in pregnancy are heartburn and constipation.
- The blood volume increases as will the red blood cell volume in pregnancy but the plasma increases out of proportion to the red blood cells so there is the perception of anemia. Even so, a woman in pregnancy can have iron deficiency anemia due to a lack of iron absorption.
- Most of the pregnancy-related reproductive system changes are directly due to the influence of estrogen and HCG on the tissues.

Quiz

1. You are explaining the cardiac changes seen in pregnancy. What can you tell the woman about her heart during pregnancy?
    a. The stroke volume decreases
    b. The cardiac output increases
    c. The heart rate decreases
    d. The chances of arrhythmia are remote

Answer: b. In pregnancy, the cardiac output, stroke volume, and heart rate all increase and there is an increased chance of a benign arrhythmia.

2. The woman is found to have an enlarged thyroid gland and an elevated total thyroxine level in the second trimester of her pregnancy. What is the next step in the evaluation?
   a. Perform a thyroid gland biopsy
   b. Obtain a radionuclide thyroid scan
   c. Obtain a total triiodothyronine level
   d. Do nothing as this is a physiological response in pregnancy

Answer: d. The pregnant patient with an enlarged thyroid gland and an elevated total thyroxine level in the second trimester of pregnancy has a normal physiological response caused by the secretion of a TSH-like hormone by the placenta.

3. What is the direct act of progesterone on the maternal respiratory status?
   a. It decreases the partial pressure of oxygen
   b. It decreases the oxygen saturation
   c. It decreases the respiratory rate
   d. It decreases the carbon dioxide level

Answer: d. Progesterone decreases the carbon dioxide level in the bloodstream and causes compensatory changes to occur in the woman's respiratory system to maintain a normal blood pH level.

4. Under what circumstances can there be an increase in kidney function in the pregnant woman?
   a. Lying on the left side
   b. Standing up
   c. Aerobically exercising
   d. Lying supine

Answer: b. Lying on the left side increases the kidney function in pregnant woman because it improves the circulation to the kidneys, increasing the amount of water filtered through the kidneys.

5. What is responsible for the skin pigment changes seen in pregnancy?
   a. Increased risk of darkening of the skin from the sun
   b. Increased keratinization of the skin tissues
   c. Increased melanocyte stimulating hormone
   d. Increased progesterone level from the placenta

Answer: c. The main thing that contributes to the pigment changes in the skin of a pregnant woman is the release of melanocyte stimulating hormone by the placenta, causing an increase in melanin production by the melanocytes of the skin.

6. If you were to draw a serum prolactin level in a woman at thirty-six weeks' gestation, what would you expect to find?
   a. A normal serum prolactin level as the patient hasn't breastfed yet
   b. A two-fold increase in prolactin level
   c. A ten-fold increase in prolactin level
   d. A one hundred-fold increase in prolactin level

Answer: c. In pregnant women at term, the serum prolactin level is increased ten-fold, which returns to normal shortly after childbirth.

7. What is the cause of peripheral edema in women who are pregnant?
    a. A decrease in the glomerular filtration rate
    b. An increase in water and salt uptake by the kidneys
    c. A decrease in serum aldosterone level
    d. An increase in serum progesterone level

Answer: b. Women in pregnancy can get peripheral edema because of an increase in water and salt uptake by the kidneys under the influence of increased aldosterone and cortisol levels, which are turned on by the placental production of corticotropin releasing hormone.

8. What is the most obvious gross anatomical change in a woman's urinary tract system during pregnancy?
    a. An enlargement of both kidneys
    b. A shrinkage of the bladder
    c. An enlargement of the ureters
    d. A foreshortening of the urethra

Answer: c. The main gross anatomical finding seen in pregnant women is hydroureter or mass enlargement of the ureters. The other changes mentioned do not occur as part of the pregnancy state.

9. What is the main factor behind the development of breast engorgement and tenderness in early pregnancy?
    a. Elevated progesterone levels
    b. Elevated HCG levels
    c. Elevated estradiol levels
    d. Elevated prolactin levels

Answer: c. Elevated estradiol levels after the woman misses her period will cause breast engorgement and tenderness that usually resolves after a few weeks' gestation.

10. Which is the main issue that leads to insulin resistance in a pregnant woman?
    a. Increased estradiol levels
    b. Increased cortisol levels
    c. Increased HCG levels
    d. Increased alkaline phosphatase levels

Answer: b. The increased cortisol levels seen in pregnancy result in an inherent insulin resistance, which can lead to gestational diabetes or frank diabetes in women who had insulin resistance prior to the pregnancy.

Chapter 4: Antepartum

Antepartum or "prenatal visits" are extremely important for the management of a healthy pregnancy and includes an initial physical exam that determines the woman's date of confinement or birth as well as the baseline status of their health. Shorter prenatal visits occur throughout the pregnancy, and for determining the status of the pregnancy and the woman's health as it relates to the pregnancy.

Pre-pregnancy Healthcare

All woman who are actively thinking about becoming pregnant seek to have the healthiest possible pregnancy. The way the doctor can help the woman do this is to plan ahead regarding the status of her health even before she thinks she might be pregnant. There are dietary and lifestyle changes that can make being pregnant a much safer option.

It should be noted that many women and their partners will be able to benefit from speaking to a healthcare provider about their intention to become pregnant. These are called pre-pregnancy or pre-conception visits. The doctor's responsibility is to take a complete history of the woman's past health problems, perform a thorough physical examination, obtain a genetic history as well as a history of diseases that run in the family. Recommendations regarding what to do to maximize the patient's ability to become pregnant will also be discussed.

Women who especially need a pre-pregnancy visit include those who have had kidney disease, diabetes, HIV disease, lupus, heart disease, hypertension, or other chronic conditions. Women who have had multiple unexplained stillbirths, children born preterm, or unexplained miscarriages will also benefit from this type of visit. Women with a recent sexually transmitted disease should be evaluated before getting pregnant. Women with an eating disorder or obesity need further evaluation prior to pregnancy. Any woman attempting to get pregnant after the age of thirty-five require pre-pregnancy counseling as well as women who have travelled to areas where the Zika virus is prevalent as this infection can cause significant fetal problems.

Prenatal Care

During prenatal care visits, the woman's vital signs are monitored, the urine is monitored for glucose and protein, and the fetal status is assessed. If there are any maternal health problems, they need to be addressed during these visits. When working with a woman who is pregnant, it is important for her to be seen as early in the pregnancy as possible to have optimal prenatal care.

The first prenatal visit tends to last much longer than other prenatal visits. The examination of the woman goes beyond an assessment of the pregnancy. There will be a complete history that needs to be obtained as well as a genetic history and a history of health problems that run in her family. Complete vital signs, including weight, height, blood pressure, pulse, and respiratory rate. A brief physical examination will likely be performed, including a thorough gynecological examination.

The main parts of the gynecological examination at the first prenatal visit includes a breast examination, looking for neoplasms or benign breast tumors, a Pap test for cervical dysplasia or the presence of human papillomavirus, and tests for chlamydia and gonorrhea, which are done by culturing the vaginal fluid. Bloodwork is drawn for a number of pregnancy and non-pregnancy-related conditions. A hemoglobin/hematocrit is drawn along with the woman's blood type. HIV testing is undertaken as well as antibody titers for rubella, syphilis, and hepatitis B. Sometimes, testing for sickle cell disease, Gaucher disease, Tay-Sachs disease, thalassemia, tuberculosis, and syphilis can be performed.

Urine testing is obtained for evidence of infection, protein in the urine, or sugar in the urine. Women who are at high risk for the Zika virus as the presence of this virus means there is a possibility of a miscarriage or fetal anomalies if the infection spreads to the fetus. Discussions are undertaken about the woman's lifestyle and personal habits that might influence the pregnancy, such as alcohol use, a smoking history, a history of an ongoing eating disorder, or a drug abuse history in the recent past. Nutritional concerns are addressed, and the woman is begun on a prenatal vitamin, which contains more folate and iron in it when compared to regular vitamins given to non-pregnant women.

There should be a discussion of exercise and diet during the first prenatal visit. The doctor should evaluate the woman's prenatal eating habits and encourage healthier habits, including eating from all food groups but not necessarily increasing the caloric content of the diet. Fetuses do not need very many calories so an increase of just one hundred calories per day is recommended and only during the last two trimesters. Exercise does not have to be restricted in pregnancy apart from contact sports.

Prenatal Visits

As most prenatal visits involve healthy women between the ages of eighteen and thirty-five, these pregnancies are usually low risk. In such cases, the first prenatal visit is done in the first trimester, followed by prenatal visits every four to six weeks until the twenty-eighth week of gestation. After this, the visits are every two weeks until the woman reaches thirty-six weeks' gestation, followed by visits every week from the thirty-sixth week of gestation until the woman delivers. Prenatal care visits should occur more often if the woman's pregnancy is high risk or if the woman's overall health is high risk.

The prenatal visit involves a shorter visit that is directed mainly at the pregnancy and involves a urine dipstick test, blood pressure evaluation, weight check, an assessment for peripheral edema, an examination of the growth of the uterus and the position of the fetus, an assessment of the fetal heartbeat, and various prenatal tests that are performed at specific intervals during the pregnancy.

Generally, a woman takes no medications other than prenatal vitamins during pregnancy. Things like aspirin, ibuprofen, herbal supplements, isotretinoin, and thalidomide are contraindicated in pregnancy. Other drugs can be taken but require specific follow up by the physician. These include certain antidepressant medications, lithium for bipolar disorder, phenytoin for seizures, fluconazole for yeast infections, albuterol for asthma, and any type of chemotherapy drug.

Prenatal testing is another big part of prenatal care. The tests are designed to follow the health of the mother and the fetus during the pregnancy. There are some tests that can tell if there is a problem with the fetus, such as testing for chromosomal anomalies or other genetic defects. The most common tests done during pregnancy to assess the mother and fetus include the one-hour glucose tolerance test, multiple marker screening, chorionic villous sampling, and amniocentesis.

Ultrasound

An ultrasound can be performed at any point in the pregnancy but is often done at about eighteen to twenty weeks to look for obvious fetal anomalies and to assess the gender of the infant. Sound waves are passed through the woman's tissue that will be converted into an image that can be identified on a bedside screen. Early ultrasounds can be done but these tend to be done for dating purposes or when there is a suspicion that either the pregnancy is not healthy or there is more than one fetus present.

The main reasons why an ultrasound is done include the conformation of the pregnancy, to assess the baby's age and growth rate, to assess the pregnancy for multiple gestation, and to determine the date of confinement. Later in the pregnancy, the ultrasound can look for obvious birth defects, such as spina bifida and heart anomalies. In the third trimester, the ultrasound can be done as part of a biophysical profile that assesses the health of the fetus in the womb.

There are a couple of different kinds of ultrasound. The type of ultrasound used depends on what is being tested and the gestational age of the fetus. In every kind of ultrasound, there is a transducer that makes us of sound waves that create a picture of the fetus on the monitor. The two most common kinds of ultrasounds are the transabdominal ultrasound and the transvaginal ultrasound. Most obstetrical ultrasounds are of the transabdominal type. The patient lies on a table and the transducer is passed across the abdomen, visualizing the fetus, the amniotic fluid, the uterus, and the ovaries. A full bladder is sometimes necessary if the uterus isn't above the level of the symphysis. The transvaginal ultrasound is done through the vagina and does not require a full bladder.

A Doppler ultrasound is done to measure the fetal heartbeat. The transducer is placed on the abdomen and picks up the flood flow through the umbilical vessels. A three-dimensional ultrasound takes thousands of pictures at the same time, making the picture of the fetus extremely lifelike and nearly as good as a picture. A four-dimensional ultrasound is similar to a three-dimensional ultrasound but differs in that it also shows fetal movements.

The ultrasound has no risks to either the woman or the fetus. It relies on sound waves rather than x-ray waves and is an excellent way of identifying problems with either the maternal pelvis, the uterus, or the fetus. It is certainly possible miss birth defects, but most birth defects can be picked up on if they are obvious to general inspection.

Figure 6 shows an ultrasound performed in the second trimester of pregnancy:

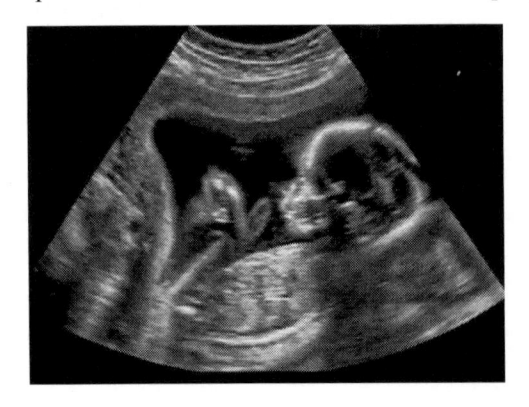

Figure 6

If an ultrasound is obtained that shows, for example, the clinical evidence of spina bifida in the female, this may be able to be treated while the baby is in utero. If the ultrasound shows the baby is breech, the option is always available to turn the baby around in what is known as external version. Cesarean sections are sometimes recommended in cases where a breech baby cannot be turned around prior to the onset of labor or when the baby is identified as being breech extremely far into the pregnancy.

The ultrasound can be done as part of a biophysical profile. It is generally performed during the third trimester to determine the health and well-being of the fetus by measuring the fetal movements, the fetal heart rate during movements, and aspects of the amniotic fluid.

Multiple Marker Screening / Quadruple

Multiple marker screening is another type of prenatal test, which is also referred to as a triple screen or a quadruple screen. It is done between fifteen and twenty weeks' gestation and is initiated with a blood draw. It can detect things like Down syndrome, spina bifida, and other fetal birth defects. The triple screen, for example, is a laboratory evaluation of the maternal alpha-fetoprotein level, the human chorionic gonadotropin level, and the unconjugated estriol level. If any of these are found to be abnormal, further studies, such as an amniocentesis can be done that will confirm the suspicions brought about as a result of the laboratory screening test.

Triple
~ hCG
~ UE3
~ MS-AFP

Chorionic Villus Sampling

This is also referred to as a CVS test. It is a prenatal test using a sampling of the tissue that attaches the fetus to the uterine wall and is normally done between the tenth and the twelfth week of pregnancy. CVS is warranted any time the maternal age is greater than thirty-five, if there are certain birth defects that run in the family, or if there is a history of a birth defect in an older sibling. The test can be done by inserting a thin tube into the cervix and collecting chorionic villus tissue. Alternatively, the woman can have a needle passed through the abdomen, trying to obtain a sample of the tissue. The main side effects of this procedure are cramping and bleeding, which are usually transitory. Infection and a spontaneous abortion are rare but possible side effects associated with this procedure.

Amniocentesis

The amniocentesis is a prenatal test that is performed more often than a chorionic villus sampling. The examiner uses an ultrasound to identify a pocket of amniotic fluid that surrounds the fetus. It takes cells that come in the amniotic fluid and checks them for chromosomal abnormalities and other problems. It can be done between fifteen weeks' and eighteen weeks' gestation. Women over the age of thirty-five have an increased need for amniocentesis as are women who have an abnormal multiple marker screening test. Anytime the woman has an older child with a major birth defect, an amniocentesis is also warranted.

The amniocentesis is done by inserting a long, thin needle through the abdominal wall, taking out a tiny amount of fluid from inside the amniotic sac. No anesthesia is necessary and rarely is there any discomfort from the procedure. The amniocentesis is extremely safe but does carry the risk of premature delivery or infection inside the uterus.

Figure 7 describes an amniocentesis:

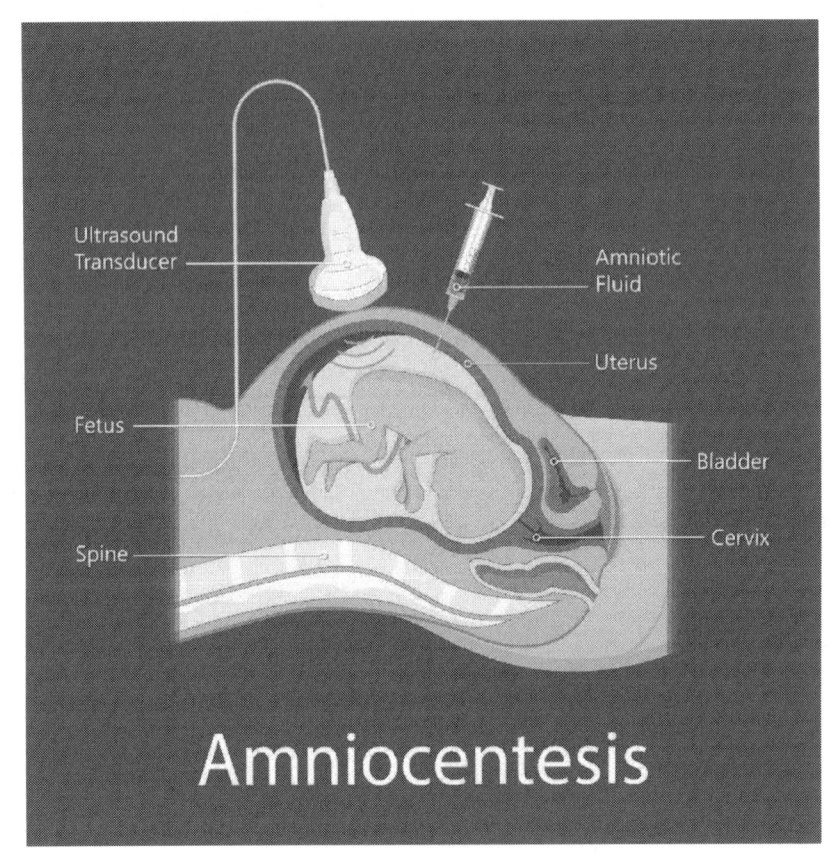

Figure 7

Gestational Diabetes Screening

Women are screened for gestational diabetes at around twenty-four weeks' gestational age. The main test offered to screen women for this disease is the one-hour glucose tolerance test. The woman can eat and drink normally prior to the test and arrives at the obstetrician's office, where she will drink a fifty-gram load of glucose in solution. Any blood sugar reading less than one hundred forty milligrams per deciliter is considered normal and no further screening or testing is necessary. If the blood sugar after a one-hour glucose tolerance test is abnormal, a three-hour glucose tolerance test is performed, which will confirm the presence or absence of gestational diabetes.

If gestational diabetes is detected, the woman will have a nutritional consultation and will follow up at the obstetrician's office more often. The woman will be monitored at home using home glucose monitoring of the blood and she will need to watch her dietary intake of carbohydrates and simple sugars. In cases where the gestational diabetes can't be controlled by diet and exercise alone, the treatment of choice is the self-administration of insulin. There are no oral medications advised for the management of gestational diabetes.

Things to Discuss

There are a variety of symptoms and health problems that come up during pregnancy that need to be discussed as part of the prenatal visit. Patients will likely complain of nausea and vomiting, heartburn, constipation, back pain, pelvic discomfort, and fatigue. These things will often be brought up by the patient but may be asked about during each prenatal visit.

Women with nausea and vomiting should be counseled to eat small portions of a bland food just prior to getting out of bed in the morning and to make use of peppermint or ginger tea. Several small meals per day should be eaten as opposed to a few larger meals. Strong spices and foods that are greasy should be avoided and fluids should be taken between meals instead of along with meals.

Heartburn can be avoided by eating several small meals per day and by avoiding larger meals that expand the stomach too much. Food should be chewed thoroughly and slowly, and the woman shouldn't not lie down immediately after eating. Clothing should be loose around the waist and the head of the bed should be elevated for sleeping at night.

Constipation should be managed as well. This can be accomplished by increasing the amount of fluids and fiber in the diet. More dried or raw fruits should be eaten as should more fresh vegetables. Bread and pasta products should be whole grain instead of refined and the woman should be encouraged to exercise.

Warning signs that indicate there might be problems with the pregnancy include sudden weight gain, particularly in the third trimester, frequent or severe headaches, facial swelling, syncope, blurry vision, pain with urination, increases in thirst, changes in the amount of urination, abnormal vaginal bleeding, and foul-smelling vaginal discharge.

Preterm labor is a more serious complication of pregnancy and occurs prior to the thirty-seventh week of pregnancy. Preterm labor is not particularly dangerous for the mother but is very dangerous for the fetus as it may be born lacking the lung maturity to breathe on its own. Typical signs of preterm labor include the presence of uterine contractions, abdominal cramping, pelvic pressure, increased vaginal discharge, leakage of amniotic fluid, vaginal bleeding, and back pain.

The Zika Virus

Women in pregnancy should know about the Zika virus. It is a virus that is particularly problematic in pregnancy, with infants born having brain dysfunction, microcephaly, and blindness. Many of the affected infants suffer from developmental delay and those that do not have birth defects run the risk of being miscarried. The virus is spread from person to person by means of mosquito bites but can be passed as a sexually transmitted disease through genital sex with an infected male. Zika primarily affects developing countries but can be seen in certain areas of the continental United States.

Key Takeaways

- Prenatal care often begins before pregnancy with a pre-pregnancy checkup to evaluate the woman's health prior to becoming pregnant.
- The first prenatal visit involves a complete history and physical examination, with determination of the date of confinement.
- Prenatal visits after the first visit are short and revolve around the growth and development of the fetus during pregnancy.
- There are several laboratory and imaging tests done during pregnancy that will help detect any abnormalities in the pregnancy and to make sure that those things that can be fixed in pregnancy are properly managed.

Quiz

1. Under what circumstances should a woman have a pre-pregnancy gynecological visit?
   a. Only if she is older than thirty-five years of age
   b. Only if she suffers from infertility
   c. Only if she has an underlying medical problem before becoming pregnant
   d. Any time a woman wants to make sure she is healthy enough for a pregnancy

Answer: d. The pre-pregnancy gynecological visit is optional but should be entertained anytime the woman wants to make sure she is healthy enough to become pregnant.

2. What blood testing is done during the first prenatal visit?
   a. Rh factor
   b. BUN and creatinine
   c. Serum albumin
   d. Gonorrhea titer

Answer: a. There are several blood tests done during the first prenatal visit. The Rh factor is one of these tests. The other tests are not done in pregnancy unless there is a specific need.

3. At which gestational age is the maternal screen for gestational diabetes performed?
   a. At the first prenatal visit
   b. Anytime sugar is found in the urine
   c. At twenty-four weeks
   d. At thirty-two weeks

Answer: c. The gestational diabetes screen is done on all pregnant women at twenty-four weeks and sooner if there is evidence to suggest the woman has gestational diabetes.

4. Preterm labor occurs prior to what gestational age?
   a. Twenty-eight weeks
   b. Thirty-two weeks
   c. Thirty-five weeks
   d. Thirty-seven weeks

Answer: d. Preterm labor is defined as any labor causing a change in the cervix prior to the thirty-seventh week of pregnancy.

5. What is not tested as part of the triple screen?
    a. Fetal karyotype
    b. Human chorionic gonadotropin
    c. Alpha fetoprotein
    d. Conjugated estriol

Answer: a. All of the above choices are evaluated as part of the triple screen with the exception of the fetal karyotype, which is not a blood test at all.

6. At which gestational age does an amniocentesis usually occur?
    a. Ten to twelve weeks
    b. Fourteen to sixteen weeks
    c. Eighteen to twenty weeks
    d. Twenty to twenty-two weeks

Answer: c. When indicated, an amniocentesis is generally performed between eighteen and twenty weeks' gestation.

7. At which gestational age is a chorionic villus sampling performed?
    a. Eight to ten weeks
    b. Ten to twelve weeks
    c. Twelve to fourteen weeks
    d. Fourteen to sixteen weeks

Answer: b. The chorionic villus sampling test is generally performed at between ten to twelve weeks' gestation.

8. In counseling a pregnant woman about her symptoms of heartburn, what do you tell her she needs to do?
    a. Take an antacid with every meal
    b. Avoid taking aspirin
    c. Elevate the head of the bed at night
    d. Eat a high protein diet

Answer: c. One thing that can be done to avoid heartburn during pregnancy is to elevate the head of the bed at night, which keeps the stomach contents from rising into the esophagus.

9. You are counseling a pregnant woman about avoiding getting the Zika virus. What do you tell her she needs to do?
    a. Avoid unwashed vegetables
    b. Avoid processed lunchmeats
    c. Avoid travel to endemic countries
    d. Avoid intercourse with anyone other than her sexual partner

Answer: c. Pregnant patients who want to avoid the Zika virus can do the most by avoiding unnecessary travel to countries where the virus is prevalent. It is passed through a mosquito bite but rarely can be passed through sexual intercourse.

10. What best describes the four-dimensional ultrasound?
    a. It gives snapshots of the fetus's structures using sound waves
    b. It gives intricate detail of the fetus's inner organs
    c. It gives realistic pictures of the fetus's facial features
    d. It combines images of the fetus and evaluates fetal movements

Answer: d. The four-dimensional ultrasound gives clear images of the fetus and evaluated fetal movements at the same time.

Chapter 5: Intrapartum

The intrapartum period of pregnancy occurs when the woman has generally reached about forty weeks' gestation and begins the process of labor and delivery. However, a fair number of women will undergo a Cesarean section, either after a failed trial of labor or as a solution to end a pregnancy where a vaginal delivery is contraindicated for fetal or maternal reasons.

Monitoring the Mother in the First Stage of Labor

Labor begins as uterine contractions begin that gradually intensify to expel the fetus and the placenta. The first stage of labor is defined as the time between the beginning of uterine contractions and the point at which the cervix is fully dilated. Most women are carefully monitored during this time for signs that may indicate a poor fetal outcome unless urgent intervention occurs. Both the condition of the mother and fetus are monitored during this stage.

An important part of the monitoring of the labor process in the first stage of labor is the partogram. This is a graph that monitors the cervical dilatation status over time. The partogram helps detect problems with cervical dilatation including a lack of progress of dilatation after several hours of what is believed to be an adequate pattern of uterine contractions.

Other things that are monitored during the first stage of labor include the mother's temperature, pulse rate, and blood pressure. The urine output is recorded, and a urinalysis is done at least once for the presence of protein and ketones, which may indicate the mother is becoming dehydrated. The general condition of the mother by observation is considered as some women will show evidence of not being able to tolerate the pain of labor and will need intervention. A woman with ongoing pain in the abdomen and pelvis between contractions require closer follow up and should be evaluated to determine the cause of significant pain. Women in the last part of the first stage of labor will become extremely restless, may suffer from vomiting, and will often have an uncontrollable urge to bear down during her contractions.

Signs that intervention is necessary include extreme anxiety, severe abdominal pain that is continuous, severe exhaustion, extreme pallor, and dehydration. Primiparous women are particularly prone to anxiety, and should be comforted and reassured that the process she is going through is normal.

Severe continuous pain in the first stage of labor usually indicates there are potential labor complications occurring including chorioamnionitis, acute pyelonephritis, systemic infection, or abruptio placentae. Rupture of the uterus can also present during this stage of labor and often presents as severe, ongoing pain.

Severe exhaustion and dehydration can occur during prolonged labor especially if the woman does not take in adequate fluids. Women with chronic anemia from iron deficiency, blood loss, or malaria can suffer from anemia and an increase in exhaustion. Bleeding from the placenta in placenta previa or abruptio placentae can increase blood loss and cause secondary weakness and exhaustion.

The woman's temperature must be continually monitored. A normal maternal temperature is between 36.0 and 37.0 degrees Celsius. The woman should have her temperature checked every four hours unless there is an indication to evaluate her temperature sooner. The temperature is recorded along with the other data on the partogram to provide a complete picture of the labor process.

When maternal fever is present, the most common causes include chorioamnionitis, pyelonephritis, or urinary tract infection. Certainly, a non-pregnancy-related illness can present with a fever and must be identified. Dehydration can also cause maternal fever. Once a source of the fever is identified, the underlying cause should be treated along with acetaminophen for fever reduction. Fever can precipitate and accelerate labor. This tends to be a more significant problem if the woman has not yet reached thirty-seven weeks' gestation.

The maternal pulse should be evaluated every two hours during the latent phase of the first stage of labor and every hour during the active phase of the first stage of labor. The normal range is between eighty and one hundred beats per minute. When it is recorded, the pulse value should be placed on the appropriate spot on the partogram. Rapid pulse rates or tachycardia can be seen with anxiety, pain, exhaustion, fever, and shock. If found to be tachycardic, the woman should be assessed for the underlying cause of the problem.

The blood pressure is also evaluated with a normal blood pressure of at least one hundred systolic and sixty diastolic or more, up to a maximum of one hundred forty systolic and ninety diastolic. The blood pressure is measured every two hours in the latent phase of labor and every hour in the active phase of labor. Hypertension can be brought on by preeclampsia or eclampsia. Hypotension can mean normal or can be secondary to pressure on the vena cava by the uterus. This is known as supine hypotension. Shock can also contribute to hypotension, which can, of course, be extremely dangerous.

The main risks of hypotension include severe kidney damage in the mother as well as maternal death if left untreated. A decrease in blood pressure may cause poor blood flow to the uterus and placenta, which reduces the fetal oxygen supply, resulting in fetal distress. If hypotension is found, the underlying cause should be identified and treated promptly. The first step is to reposition the mother from the supine position to the left-lying position. Any hemorrhage should be quickly reversed with blood products and crystalloid solution.

Shock should be differentiated from hypotension. Shock involves hypotension and tachycardia with cold skin that is diaphoretic. Shock in the first stage of labor is almost exclusively due to hemorrhage from placenta previa or placental abruption. A ruptured uterus is a secondary cause of shock. Infection is another cause of shock that can be identified.

The urine should be monitored for the volume, the presence of proteins, and the presence of ketones. This can be assessed by periodically putting a dipstick in a sample of urine. It needs to be done every four hours in the latent phase of labor and every two hours in the active stage of labor. If the woman voids before this time, the urine should also be tested. The observations need to be recorded on the partogram. Remember that women given IV fluids containing glucose in labor will have a positive dipstick for glucose and this doesn't mean she is diabetic or in any danger to her fetus after birth.

Women with a urine output of less than twenty milliliters per hour are considered oliguric. Oliguria can be seen in dehydration, shock, and severe pre-eclampsia. If these conditions are present, a continual observation of the urine should be undertaken by means of an indwelling urinary catheter. The cause of the poor urine output needs to be determined and adequate hydration provided by intravenous or oral means. If a cesarean section is planned, all fluids must be by intravenous means.

Proteinuria on a dipstick above trace findings is not a normal phenomenon. It generally signifies preeclampsia during labor but can indicate a urinary tract infection or kidney disease. The woman with proteinuria should be evaluated for a urinary tract infection. Any urine dipstick with two plus protein should be seen as having chronic renal disease or preeclampsia. Ketonuria, on the other hand, is common in labor but can be a sign of exhaustion that should be addressed.

Women who are exhausted will not generally have a good outcome and it can manifest itself as fetal distress secondary to hypoxia. It can be prevented by giving adequate oral or intravenous fluids, such as Ringer's lactate with five percent dextrose. Pain also needs to be controlled to fight exhaustion. Any steps that can be taken to shorten the labor should be undertaken. Fifty percent dextrose solution should be avoided as this can be bad for the fetus.

Monitoring the Fetus in the First Stage of Labor

It is crucial to monitor the fetus during labor as this can have an extremely positive effect on fetal outcome. Labor necessarily puts added stress on the fetus and, while most fetuses tolerate this stress, in some infants the stress becomes "distress" requiring intervention. The most common cause of stress in labor is head compression, which is completely normal.

Decreases in oxygen supply to the fetus is a more ominous cause of fetal stress. Extended labor with cephalopelvic disproportion can mean ongoing head compression and this type of fetal distress can become problematic due to its long duration. Uterine contractions alone can cause fetal distress and fetal hypoxia because of decreased available oxygen supply to the fetus. In fact, uterine contractions are the most common cause of fetal hypoxia in labor. Abnormal uterine blood vessels can make this problem worse.

The placenta may be old and may fail to allow enough oxygen to get to the fetus. Preeclampsia contributes to placental insufficiency by adversely affecting the vessels and blood supply to the placenta. Maternal smoking can also narrow the uterine blood vessels, resulting in fetal hypoxia. Abruptio placentae or partial separation of the placenta from the uterine wall can cause hypoxia by tearing way the vessels that normally supply the fetus. Cord prolapse or cord compression directly block blood flow to the placenta, resulting in fetal distress.

The response of the fetus to hypoxia can be determined. A decrease in the normal blood oxygen concentration is the definition of hypoxia. If hypoxia isn't very severe, the fetus adjusts and will have no change in heart rate. With further hypoxia, late decelerations of the heartbeat rate can be seen after a contraction. This can be followed by fetal bradycardia independent of a contraction, while severe fetal hypoxia may lead to fetal death.

The two main ways to evaluate the presence of fetal hypoxia are to do continuous fetal monitoring by external Doppler readings or with an internal scalp electrode. The finding of meconium-stained amniotic fluid is also a sign of fetal hypoxia. If the determination is made not to evaluate a fetus continuously as the pregnancy is considered low-risk, intermittent Doppler monitoring of the heartrate should be done, particularly during and shortly after the contraction. The heart tones should be monitored every two hours during the latent phase of labor and every half hour during the active phase of labor (at a minimum).

Three main things should be evaluated in regards to the fetal heartrate. The baseline rate should be determined and should be between one hundred ten and one hundred sixty. The beat-to-beat variability should be monitored, which is a sign of fetal health and wellbeing. The presence of accelerations and decelerations should be noted. Accelerations with movement portend a good outcome and indicates the fetus has enough oxygen to move about.

Decelerations are reductions in heartrate that can be normal if they happen during head compression or at the same time as the contraction. These are called early decelerations. Decelerations are abnormal if they follow the contraction, in which case they are caused late decelerations. Another normal deceleration is a variable deceleration that involves sporadic decelerations unrelated to a contraction.

A loss of beat-to-beat variation in the heartbeat is also a sign of fetal distress. Any time there is a flat tracing on the fetal monitor, this should be taken seriously as a sign of fetal distress. It can also mean the fetus is asleep or has received IV analgesia from the mother. All findings should be considered with the clinical picture in mind. A sleeping baby can always be awakened with gentle external pressure on the uterus and should restore beat-to-beat variability.

Baseline tachycardia should also be taken seriously. A baseline fetal heartrate of more than one hundred sixty beats per minute carries some meaning. It can be from fever in the mother, maternal exhaustion, chorioamnionitis, fetal anemia, fetal hemorrhage, or the administration of certain drugs to the mother that increase the fetal heart rate. The chance of fetal distress is higher with fetal tachycardia. This is especially true of tachycardia associated with decelerations.

Baseline bradycardia stems from a fetal heartbeat of less than one hundred. The main cause of this finding is fetal distress secondary to fetal hypoxia. If decelerations are also present, it means there is likely life-threatening fetal distress.

In cases of obvious fetal distress, fetal resuscitation in utero should be undertaken. It first involves placing the mother on her side and giving her one hundred percent oxygen by mask. An IV with Ringer's lactate should be given to bring the mothers' fluid volume up and every attempt should be made to deliver the baby as soon as possible. If the cervix is dilated, forceps or a vacuum extractor should be used to deliver the fetus vaginally. If an imminent vaginal delivery is not possible, an emergency Cesarean section needs to take place. In unusual cases, intravenous terbutaline can be given, which slow the rate of contractions, allowing for a period of rest and recovery for the woman and fetus.

About ten to twenty percent of vaginal deliveries result in meconium staining of the amniotic fluid. It is much more common among women in the forty-second week of gestation or later. Thin meconium staining is different from thick meconium staining. Thinly stained amniotic fluid tends not to be as severe as thick meconium amniotic fluid. It usually means there has been fetal hypoxia in the past or ongoing fetal hypoxia. If there is no other evidence of fetal hypoxia, nothing needs to be done about the meconium staining until birth, when it is suctioned out of the trachea to prevent meconium aspiration syndrome.

Monitoring the Labor Progress

A woman is considered in labor when she has regular uterine contractions about every ten minutes apart with a change in cervical dilatation or effacement or the presence of ruptured membranes. The two main stages of this part of labor include the latent and the active phase. The latent phase is first and goes from no cervical dilatation to three centimeters' dilatation. With first-time moms, the cervix also needs to be fully effaced before the next phase of labor commences. Multigravidas may enter the active phase without full cervical effacement. The latent phase lasts no longer than eight hours in normal labor. The contractions intensify during this phase and get longer.

The active phase results in more rapid cervical dilatation, and more frequent and prolonged contractions. It is expected that the cervix should dilate about one centimeter an hour, but this can be highly variable and one centimeter per hour represents the lowest acceptable dilatation progression.

Upon admission to the labor and delivery unit, the mother should have a brief physical examination to assess her overall health and an evaluation of the status of her labor should be determined. The partogram is filled out as the labor progresses, which can tell how the labor is progressing and what other findings have been gathered in assessing the fetus and the mother. A complete maternal evaluation and examination should be done every four hours, regardless of where she is in the laboring process.

If it is determined that the progress of labor is slower than expected and especially if the woman is tiring, the doctor may induce or augment the woman's labor. Sometimes, rupturing the membranes in the latent phase can bring on active labor. If the woman is HIV positive or if contractions are poor, intravenous oxytocin may be administered. These women need more stepped up physical evaluations at shorter intervals than just every four hours. Women with HIV should have artificial rupture of membranes as late as possible to avoid maternal transmission of the virus to the infant.

If a woman spontaneously ruptures her membranes during labor, the doctor may have to intervene. If the head is palpable four fifths above the pubic symphysis or the infant is breech, there is a high likelihood of cord prolapse, which must be monitored for. If the head is three fifths or less above the pubic symphysis and vertex, the chances of a cord prolapse are much less. Even so, the fetus's heart rate should be monitored regularly for evidence of cord compression or fetal distress. Upon rupture of membranes, an assessment of meconium staining should be undertaken to plan for the delivery and to have a higher index of suspicion for fetal distress in labor.

Poor progression in labor can be from any one of four things, known as the "four P's". The first P is the "patient". Is her pain managed? If not, she may be holding back and adversely affecting the contractions. Is she anxious? This can slow the labor process and she may need emotional support. Is the bladder full? This can prevent the dropping of the head into the pelvic brim. Is the patient dehydrated? Hydration is necessary to have adequately strong contractions. If so, IV fluids may need to be given.

The second P is "powers". This means that labor can be halted if the power of the contractions is ineffective to bring about cervical dilatation. Inadequate uterine contractions can be too short in duration, too far apart, or too weak in intensity. If they last less than forty seconds per contraction or if there are less than two contractions per minute, these are ineffective contractions. In some cases, these things are met but the actual force of the contractions is less than adequate. These are called dysfunctional uterine contractions and things like oxytocin and an intrauterine pressure catheter need to be placed to enhance the strength of the contractions.

The third P is the "passenger". The infant may be in an abnormal position or may be too large to enter the birth canal. There isn't an adequate amount of pressure on the cervix by the fetal presenting part and this causes slow cervical dilatation. If the fetal lie is anything other than longitudinal and cephalic, the only option may be to halt the labor and progress to a Cesarean section.

The fourth P is "passage". This can adversely affect the progress of labor because the birth canal is too narrow or is not of a gynecoid shape, which would make a vaginal birth more difficult. If the membranes are intact with a narrow pelvis, they should be ruptured and the mother should be allowed to labor an additional four hours before a diagnosis of "poor progress" can be made. Excessive fetal molding along with a high presenting part indicates a small pelvis and may mean there is enough cephalopelvic disproportion, necessitating a Cesarean section.

Overall, the two main causes of poor progression in labor are cephalopelvic disproportion and inadequate uterine contractions. Inadequate uterine contractions are almost exclusively seen in primiparas and can be fixed with intravenous oxytocin. If cephalopelvic disproportion is the problem despite rupture of membranes, the answer is to have a consult for a Cesarean section.

Cord prolapse can happen at any time in the labor process and is a serious complication of labor because it abruptly blocks the blood supply to the fetus with each contraction. For the cord to be truly prolapse, the membranes have to be ruptured. If they are not ruptured, the cord is said to be the presenting part but is not prolapsed. A cord prolapse is an automatic indication for an emergency Cesarean section. The only exception is the presence of prolapsed cord at nine to ten centimeters' cervical dilatation, where the infant can be quickly delivered vaginally.

Examining the Vagina in Labor

Women in labor need regular vaginal exams to assess the cervical dilatation status and the presenting part. There should always be equipment ready at the bedside for a sterile vaginal examination, even if the membranes haven't obviously ruptured. Sterile gloves, swabs, and tap water are necessary, as is a sterile instrument that can be used to rupture the membranes. An antiseptic vaginal cream or sterile water-based ointment is used to lubricate the sterile gloves. The woman is placed supine with her knees up and the examiner inserts two lubricated, gloved fingers into the vagina. The two fingers are used to identify the cervix and estimate the degree to which it has dilated.

If the woman is suspected of having rupture of membranes without labor, a speculum exam should be done first to take a swab of the fluid coming from the cervix. The swab is twirled on a slide and the slide is quickly dried. The microscope slide is then placed under low power in the laboratory with an assessment made as to whether ferning pattern can be seen on the dried secretions. Only amniotic fluid will yield this ferning pattern so that it can help define whether the membranes have ruptured. After this is shown, a gloved vaginal examination can take place.

During the examination, the diameter of the cervical os is determined in centimeters by estimation. Effacement is determined by estimating the thickness of the cervical outlet. It is measured as zero percent effacement if it is about two centimeters in thickness and is measured as one hundred percent effacement if the cervix is extremely thin. The presenting part is determined during this examination and usually sutures can be felt, which determine the exact position of the fetal head. Estimations as to the degree to which the head has descended into the pelvic inlet can be made this way, but it isn't as good as doing an abdominal assessment of how much head remains above the pubic symphysis. Upon withdrawal of the gloved hand, blood, amniotic fluid characteristics, and meconium staining can be determined.

Managing the Partogram

The partogram is part graph and part a descriptive document. It is maintained throughout the labor process to identify the progression of labor and to quickly determine any changes or red flags that need to be evaluated as part of the monitoring of the first stage of labor. The assessment of the mother is performed and recorded on the partogram. The assessment of the fetus is also performed and recorded on the partogram. The progress of the labor is the final thing recorded on the partogram.

When evaluating the mother, there should be regular measurements of her vital signs, including her pulse, blood pressure, and temperature. The urinary volume needs to be recorded in milliliters and dipstick readings for protein and ketones are qualitatively given. Any drugs given to the mother, including IV fluids can be listed on the partogram.

The fetal heart rate pattern is noted on the partogram, particularly the baseline heart rate and the presence or absence of decelerations. If decelerations are found, the type of deceleration needs to be recorded. If meconium staining is present, this should be noted. The cervical dilatation status is recorded over time as well as the effacement. Aspects of the presenting part are also recorded, including the presenting part, the position of the presenting part, and the presence or absence of molding. Molding can be graded according to its severity. The duration of the contractions and the length of time between contractions should also be documented.

Second Stage of Labor

The second stage of labor is from the moment the cervix opens to ten centimeters' dilation or fully dilated and ends with the expulsion of the fetus. Typical signs and symptoms of the second stage of labor include extremely intense contractions that are very close together. The patient has an increase in restlessness and may suffer nausea and vomiting. Most patients have an uncontrollable urge to bear down or push the baby out. The perineum begins to bulge during the contraction as it is being stretched by the presenting part of the fetus. If the patient is exhibiting signs of being in the second stage of labor, an abdominal and vaginal examination should take place to determine if the woman can begin to push. Primigravidas usually have an engaged head at the start of the second stage of labor; however, many multiparas do not have an engaged head but have a fully dilated cervix. The head is considered engaged when only two-fifths of the head is above the pubic symphysis and the largest transverse diameter of the head has already passed below the pelvic inlet.

Figure 8 shows the different stages of labor and delivery:

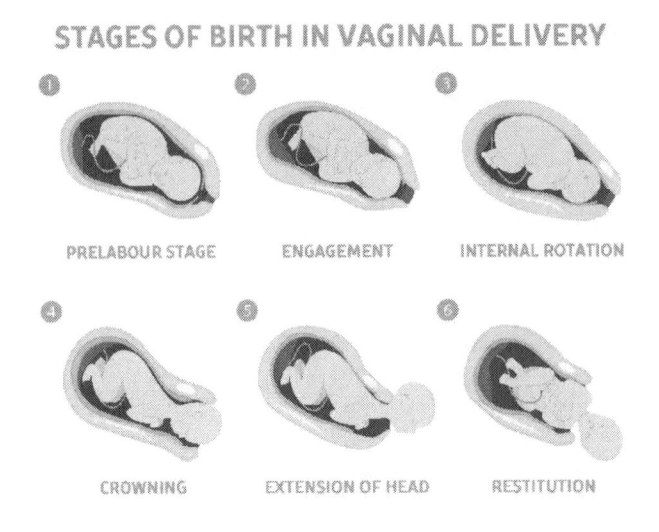

STAGES OF BIRTH IN VAGINAL DELIVERY

PRELABOUR STAGE — ENGAGEMENT — INTERNAL ROTATION

CROWNING — EXTENSION OF HEAD — RESTITUTION

Figure 8

While some practitioners advise pushing as soon as the cervix is ten centimeters dilated. Others recommend waiting until the head is bulging at the perineum as this will yield the strongest urge to push and make pushing more effective. Overall, either method is appropriate if the woman is tolerating the contractions and there is no evidence of fetal distress or cephalopelvic disproportion. If the decision is made to wait, the woman needs to be assessed every hour for evidence of engagement of the fetal head.

The main difference between the first and the second stage of labor is the involvement of the mother in the process. She needs to be extremely physically active in the second stage of labor as contractions alone will not likely deliver the baby. The woman who efficiently uses her strength will have the best possible outcome with the shortest second stage. Resting can occur between contractions although they tend to occur with greater frequency than is seen in the first stage of labor. One long pushing effort is preferred over several short pushes per contraction.

Assisted deliver with forceps or vacuum extraction needs to be done if the second stage of labor does not progress. If a primigravida has inadequate contractions and doesn't have obvious cephalopelvic disproportion, she is a candidate for an assisted delivery or intravenous oxytocin if the contractions to don't seem to be effective enough. If cephalopelvic disproportion is increasingly evident, then a cesarean section is probably the only option. The same is true for primiparas who have evidence of fetal distress and have longer than a few minutes before the delivery of the fetus. An episiotomy should be done in any second-stage fetal distress situation as this greatly speeds the time of delivery. The bladder can be emptied with an indwelling urinary catheter to make the most room possible for rapid delivery of the infant.

Figure 9 shows typical forceps used in pregnancy and delivery:

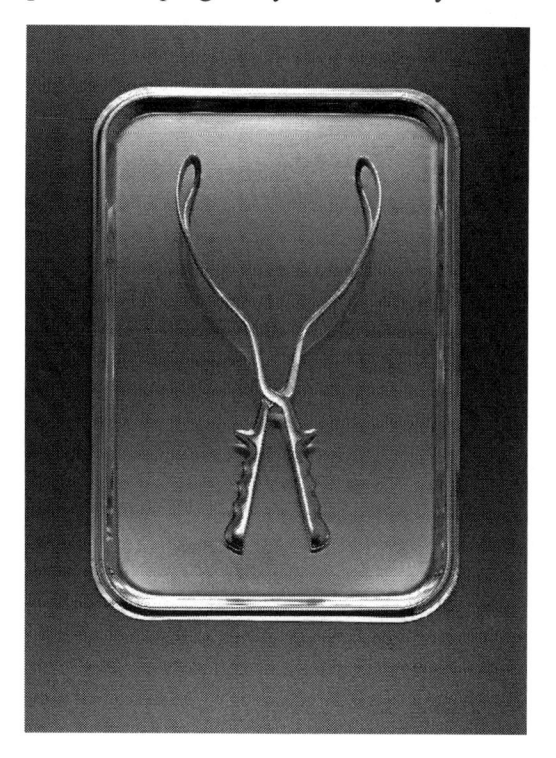

Figure 9

Near the end of the second stage, the head crowns in the vaginal outlet. If tearing is expected, an episiotomy is performed to prevent a more difficult to treat laceration. A hand is placed on the infant's vertex and another hand on the perineum to guide the head out. The cord, if present, should be removed from around the baby's neck and the head is rotated to one side. The anterior shoulder is delivered first, and this is followed by the delivery of the posterior shoulder. The rest of the baby will generally slip out unaided.

Episiotomies are no longer routinely performed but there are indications for still doing them in certain circumstances. If the infant is in distress, an episiotomy is performed, and when the woman will likely lacerate the perineum, an episiotomy is performed. Prolonged second stages with maternal exhaustion are often helped by doing an episiotomy. Women with a thick perineum or a previous third or fourth degree tear should have an episiotomy. Women who had a previous rectocele repair need an episiotomy. Second degree tears, however, heal faster than an episiotomy so, if just a second-degree tear is expected, no episiotomy needs to be done.

Median or midline episiotomies are the most common procedures performed. The cut is made from the vagina down the midline of the perineum that is about an inch long and that doesn't extend to the rectum. Mediolateral episiotomies can be done if the midwife or obstetrician has more experience with mediolateral repair.

A prolonged second stage can be defined in a couple of ways. If a primigravida can bear down for more than forty-five minutes and if a multigravida bears down for more than thirty minutes without delivery of the infant, this is known as a prolonged second stage. The doctor must be in attendance by this time and the woman should be given options regarding assisted delivery with vacuum extraction or forceps. If cephalopelvic disproportion is present or if there is fetal distress, the choice of an assisted delivery is secondary and the need for a Cesarean section is primary.

Dealing with Shoulder Dystocia

Sometimes, the head is delivered successfully but the shoulders will not fit out of the pelvic inlet. Patients at the greatest risk for this are women with large infants, women with gestational diabetes, and women who are obese. The first clue to this being the case is a prolonged second stage that ends with a large fetal head with fat cheeks. The head doesn't rotate normally after exiting the vagina and the shoulders become stuck. Maneuvers to turn the fetus are often difficult and may not work. An assistant must push on the suprapubic area while the obstetrician moves the woman to the edge of the table so that more range can be obtained by posteriorly flexing the neck. However, too much traction can cause brachial plexus palsy so this should be done gently. The goal is to get the anterior shoulder to pass underneath the symphysis while the mother is bearing down as strongly as she can. Once the anterior shoulder is delivered, the posterior shoulder generally comes next. These maneuvers are collectively called the MacRobert's method of delivering a shoulder dystocia.

The Episiotomy

There are two different types of episiotomies. These include the mediolateral or oblique episiotomy and the midline episiotomy. The midline episiotomy is technically more difficult and runs the risk of extending into the rectal muscles or the rectal mucosa as a third-degree tear or fourth-degree tear, respectively. A mediolateral episiotomy is done when the presenting part is bulging out of the perineum but is not expected to arrive with an intact perineum. During the height of the contraction, an incision is made at a forty-five-degree angle away from the anus, usually on the left side. Two fingers are placed between the fetal head and the perineum so that the fetus isn't injured by the cut. When the procedure is done late in the second stage of labor, the amount of bleeding is minimal as the head is providing some hemostasis.

After the delivery of the child, the perineum is anesthetized topically unless epidural anesthesia is in place. Absorbable sutures approximate the damaged muscles and connective tissue, with the final sutures placed in a running fashion to close the skin. At no time should non-absorbable sutures be placed as they are extremely uncomfortable and require removal.

The Third Stage of Labor

The third stage of labor is often overlooked as it is usually the shortest stage of labor and is somewhat anti-climactic after the delivery of the infant. It begins once the infant has been delivered and ends when the placenta is safely removed from the uterus. The average length of this stage of labor is only about three to five minutes but it can be up to thirty minutes. Uterine contractions continue during this stage as it tries to expel a placenta that is no longer necessary. The uterine size shrinks and dislodges the placenta so that it can be gently pulled with traction to remove it in its entirety. The uterine contractions slow the bleeding process and clotting occurs inside the uterus.

The most common complication of the third stage of labor is excessive bleeding so this can be a very dangerous time for the mother. Postpartum hemorrhage remains the most common cause of maternal death among women in developing countries. Selectively managing the third stage by pressing on the uterus and putting gentle traction on the placenta will decrease the total amount of bleeding as opposed to passively waiting for the placenta to deliver spontaneously. Oxytocin is then given to contract the uterus further. Nevertheless, some midwives prefer the passive method of delivering the placenta.

After delivery of the placenta, it should be inspected. The placentas should be evaluated for completeness and to make sure there are no cotyledons left in the uterus. The membranes must be attached to the placenta with a round hole where the fetus passed through. Cloudy membranes or tissue that smells badly might suggest an ongoing chorioamnionitis necessitating intervention. Clots on the cotyledons suggest that there may have been a partial abruption before birth. Placental infarcts will be identified as being firm and pale in appearance when compared to the blood red color of the normal placenta. There are two arteries and one vein in the umbilical cord, and these should be examined. The placenta should be weighed and should be about four hundred fifty to six hundred fifty grams at full term. Heavy placentas are suggestive of congenital syphilis. Heavy and pale placentas suggest Rh disease. Maternal diabetes also creates a heavy placenta. Lighter placentas are found in infants that are small for gestational age.

If the placenta has not been delivered within thirty minutes, this is called a prolonged third stage of labor. If the active method of extraction has failed, oxytocin intravenously should be given to try and increase the intrauterine pressure so the placenta can be expelled. If only the umbilical cord can be seen entering the cervix, it is considered "retained". The patient runs the risk of having postpartum hemorrhage during this time and requiring the patient to be taken to the operating suite and surgically removing the placenta under controlled intraoperative conditions and general anesthesia.

Management of Postpartum Hemorrhage

Postpartum hemorrhage is defined as losing more than five hundred milliliters of blood within the first twenty-four hours after a vaginal or operative delivery. If the bleeding is occurring while the placenta is still in the uterus, the patient needs oxytocin and active attempts to remove the placenta though pressure on the fundus and gentle traction on the cord. If this doesn't cause extraction of the placenta, the only real option is to perform an intraoperative placental extraction.

If the bleeding happens after the placenta has been delivered, this can be extremely dangerous. Oxytocin, blood products, and IV fluids must be given urgently to control the atony of the uterus and replace lost fluids and blood products. Attempts to contract the uterus using a bimanual examination should also be undertaken. Uterine massage should be done on an ongoing basis. The bladder needs to be emptied as this can impair the process of trying to get the uterus to contract. Aortic compression is a last-ditch effort to slow the flow of blood to the uterus. Remember that atony is not the only cause of a postpartum hemorrhage and that trauma to the cervix or uterus during the birth process can also affect bleeding. These types of problems may need operative intervention.

The main causes of a postpartum hemorrhage that must be considered include: 1) blood clots in the uterus; 2) uterine atony; 3) retained placental cotyledons; 4) prolonged first stage of labor; 5) large infant; 6) multiple gestation pregnancy; 7) full bladder; 8) use of oxytocin in labor; 9) general anesthesia use; 10) placental abruption; and 11) polyhydramnios.

Analgesia in Intrapartum Care

While some women choose to have no anesthesia or analgesia during the labor and delivery process, others cannot tolerate the pain and will need some type of pain relief. Pain relief is not the same as sedation or anesthesia. Ideally, a pain-relieving drug in labor will affect the sensation of pain without causing drowsiness. General anesthesia is rarely used in labor and delivery and is reserved for extremely urgent cesarean sections and the operative removal of the placenta.

In the United States, epidural anesthesia is extremely popular. In such cases, the anesthetist places a catheter in the lumbar region of the woman's spinal column and pumps a steady dose of Fentanyl or morphine into the epidural space, allowing for movement but severely restricting the patient's perception of pain. The biggest advantage of epidural anesthesia is that it can be used for episiotomy repair and for a Cesarean section, should one urgently be required during the labor process.

Opiates can be given by intravenous or intramuscular routes, but these are usually done earlier in the first stage when it will be expected to wear off at the time of delivery. Failure of this to happen may result in a baby that is floppy and has a poor respiratory drive because of opiate sedation. Other places make use of nitrous oxide as an inhalational analgesic. Promethazine and hydroxyzine are given for control of nausea and will relax the woman. Naloxone must be on hand for both the mother and the infant if opiates are used to achieve analgesia.

There is no role for benzodiazepines or barbiturates in labor. While they may relax the woman, they offer nothing in the way of pain relief and only sedate both the mother and the infant. They are also more difficult to reverse with an antidote should too much medication be given. On the other hand, women who want to avoid injections during labor might do well by inhaling a mixture of nitrous oxide and oxygen, which provides brief respite from the pain of labor and is completely safe to use in the labor and delivery process.

After delivery, there is generally no need for any parenteral anesthesia or analgesia. If an episiotomy needs to be repaired, one percent xylocaine is used to anesthetize the perineal and vaginal tissues locally to allow for a relatively pain-free way of repairing the tears and lacerations. This is generally extremely safe, although using too much of it has been known to increase the seizure threshold and cause seizures.

Key Takeaways

- Intrapartum care involves the care of the woman in labor from the time of the first contractions to the delivery of the placenta.
- The goal is to have a normal vaginal delivery; however, due to modern techniques that can predict a difficult vaginal delivery, there are many cesarean sections done, even on women who haven't had a trial of labor.

- The first stage of labor is monitored by the nurse, who records all the vital data on the patient and the fetus on a partogram.
- The second stage of labor begins when the cervix is fully dilated and ends with the expulsion of the fetus.
- The third stage of labor begins when the infant is born and ends when the placenta is expelled.
- After delivery of the placenta, any tears, lacerations, or episiotomies are repaired and postpartum bleeding is controlled.

Quiz

1. The woman being seen in labor is six centimeters dilated and is having a slowing of her contractions. What initial step can be taken that will increase the rate of her contractions?
    a. Have her sit on the toilet
    b. Perform an amniotomy
    c. Add IV fluids to her treatment plan
    d. Apply prostaglandin E2 gel to the cervix

Answer: b. An amniotomy will break the bag of water which generally stimulate contractions, particularly in the active phase of the first stage of labor.

2. Why is it not a good idea to perform an amniotomy in the latent phase of labor in an HIV-infected mother?
    a. It will increase her bleeding risk.
    b. It increases the chance of getting chorioamnionitis.
    c. It tends not to increase the strength and frequency of her contractions.
    d. It increases the fetus's exposure to the HIV virus in utero.

Answer: d. An amniotomy should be done late in labor or not at all in HIV-infected mothers as doing so provides a longer period for the fetus to be exposed to the maternal blood and to potentially contract HIV as a neonate.

3. A woman is being evaluated in the first stage of labor. What clinical finding warrants further investigation?
    a. A sudden gush of clear fluid from the vagina
    b. A maternal temperature of 99.0 degrees Fahrenheit
    c. Continuous abdominal pain
    d. Increased urinary frequency

Answer: c. Continuous abdominal pain is not normal in the first stage of labor and might mean chorioamnionitis or an abrupted placenta. This finding needs further intervention.

4. The doctor is preparing to perform an episiotomy. What is the main advantage of doing a mediolateral episiotomy?
    a. It is technically easier to do
    b. The blood loss is less
    c. There is less pain with this type of episiotomy

d. There is no chance of extension into the rectum

Answer: a. The main advantage of a mediolateral episiotomy is that it is technically easier to do. The blood loss can be more with this type and the pain is often greater. It still has the potential to extend into the rectum but to a lesser degree than is true of a midline episiotomy.

5. You are evaluating a woman prior to labor who you suspect will have shoulder dystocia. What things might lead you to be prepared for this problem in the second stage of labor?
    a. Previous baby weighing nine pounds
    b. Gestational diabetes
    c. Onset of labor at thirty-seven weeks
    d. Male gender of fetus

Answer: b. Women with gestational diabetes often have very large babies and put themselves at risk of having shoulder dystocia during the second stage of her labor.

6. For what reason might the doctor choose to tell the laboring woman to wait on pushing in the second stage until there is bulging of the perineum?
    a. Pushing too early can lead to fetal distress
    b. Pushing late in the second stage provides less blood loss
    c. Pushing late in the second stage provides for more effective pushing
    d. The baby will be delivered just as quickly if she waits

Answer: c. Some doctors choose to have the woman wait to push until the perineum is bulging, which is associated with a stronger urge to push and more effective pushing.

7. The woman is in the third stage of labor. What is the most common cause of bleeding in this stage of labor?
    a. Retained placenta or placental fragments
    b. Uterine laceration
    c. Cervical laceration
    d. Full bladder

Answer: a. The most common cause of bleeding in the third stage of labor is a retained placenta or retained placental fragments.

8. What is the main purpose of the partogram?
    a. To document the mother's vital signs
    b. To document the mother's urine output
    c. To keep track of the fetal heart tracing
    d. To mark cervical dilatation status over time

Answer: d. The partogram has many features but its main purpose is to document the cervical dilatation status over time and to detect things like a prolonged labor or precipitous labor.

9. The doctor is managing a woman who has sustained a postpartum hemorrhage. What does this mean?
    a. She has lost blood after the delivery of the placenta
    b. She required blood transfusions after the delivery

c. She lost more than 500 milliliters of blood in twenty-four hours
   d. She required intraoperative intervention to control bleeding

Answer: c. The basic definition of a postpartum hemorrhage is having lost 500 milliliters of blood within the first twenty-four hours after childbirth. It can be from many causes.

10. In examining the placenta, you see a firm blood clot on the side of the placenta that had been attached to the uterine wall. What can you surmise from this?
    a. The patient has a cotyledon left in the placenta
    b. The woman has normal clotting factors and doesn't have a bleeding disorder
    c. She had an area of placental infarction near term
    d. She had a partially abrupted placenta near term

Answer: d. The patient with a blood clot adherent to the placenta likely had a partial abruption at the time of labor or shortly before going into labor.

Chapter 6: Postpartum

The postpartum or puerperium period begins as soon as the woman gives birth and technically ends at about six weeks after the birth of the child. Some problems of the postpartum state do not manifest themselves until after the six-week mark. The obstetrician must be aware of this and should consider the possibility that a postpartum woman may need care even after a six-week postpartum visit.

Postpartum Care in the Hospital

The postpartum period is also known as the puerperium, which is the time between the delivery of the placenta and the time it takes for the woman's body and mind to return to normal. This period is different for every woman but the average time suggested by most experts is six weeks. Even so, it can take many months for some of the pregnant woman's body systems to become completely normal again. Things like the perineum never return to the state they were in when the woman was pregnant as the area was completely stretched out during childbirth. As part of the postpartum visit at six weeks after the birth, it is the job of the doctor or midwife to determine if the woman has, indeed, returned to her pre-pregnancy state. During this time, vast changes in the woman's mental and emotional state may occur.

The puerperium is when the woman begins the process of breastfeeding her infant and makes decisions regarding what kind of birth control she needs. Almost every organ system undergoes some type of change during this period. Right after birth, the new mother will begin shivering even though her body temperature hasn't changed. The pulse rate and blood pressure are monitored to make sure the levels aren't too low or too high. The new mother will lose weight immediately after giving birth and on average, will lose eight kilograms instantly. As the uterus shrinks in the next few weeks, she will lose even more weight and produce extra urine as she eliminates the extra fluid that was necessary during pregnancy.

The skin changes that occurred during pregnancy will not normalize as quickly, and the areas that were darkened during pregnancy will remain dark for many months to come. The puffiness in the face and the swelling of the ankles will recede in a brief period. There will be an increase in sweating in the days following the birth. The abdominal wall will be flaccid after the delivery and there may be separation of the abdominal musculature. Any stretch marks developed during pregnancy gradually become less red over time. Some women become extremely hungry while others are extremely anorexic. There is often an increase in flatulence. Painful hemorrhoids and pain from an episiotomy, when performed, may both contribute to the woman becoming constipated.

Some women experience urinary retention after the birth of their child because of swelling of the urethra during the childbirth experience. After the swelling goes down, the woman often experiences diuresis starting two to three days after the delivery. If the woman is edematous during pregnancy, she may have an increase in urinary output immediately after birth. Some women experience stress incontinence during periods of coughing and laughing. It may begin soon after delivery or may be a continuation of the stress incontinence she experienced as a pregnant woman. Stress incontinence may become worse shortly after birth but gets better as the pelvic floor muscles strengthen.

The woman's hemoglobin begins to stabilize around the fourth day after birth. The platelet count becomes elevated and the platelets have an increase in coagulability, which puts the postpartum woman at a higher than average risk of having a thromboembolic event. There may be significant changes in the breast tissue, particularly if the woman breastfeeds. The breasts begin producing milk within a few days of delivery and continue to produce milk if they are stimulated by the suckling of the infant. The vulva is extremely swollen and congested shortly after delivery but quickly shrinks back to its normal size. Any lacerations or episiotomies are quickly healed in the perineum and rarely become infected or fail to resolve. Small vaginal tears generally heal in seven to ten days.

Women who have never given birth before have an external os that is circular in their cervix but, after the first pregnancy, this os becomes shaped like a slit. The vagina is quite enlarged after birth, but shrinks rapidly so that it returns to have normal rugae by the third postpartum week. The vaginal walls never, however, shrink to a pre-pregnancy size and there is an increased chance of vaginal prolapse in the form of a cystocele or a rectocele. The cervix doesn't close right away but closes a week after the birth. The uterus rapidly involutes but doesn't reach a normal size until about six weeks' postpartum.

Shortly after birth, the uterus is about the size of a uterus at twenty weeks' gestation. By the end of the first week, it will have shrunk down to the level of a twelve-week gestation uterus. By two weeks, the uterus is no longer palpable above the pubic symphysis. Even though the uterus shrinks maximally by the sixth postpartum week, it never shrinks down to the size of a normal non-pregnant uterus. The inner lining of the uterus dies off secondary to ischemia and leaves the uterus in what is known as the lochia. Red lochia lasts twenty-four days and then becomes the color of straw. It should be noted that the normal lochia has a slight smell but it is not malodorous. Malodorous lochia usually signifies an infection.

The puerperium begins when the placenta is delivered. The woman rests in the hospital for a day or two and then goes home with over-the-counter pain medications. She is seen at six-weeks' postpartum during which she is re-examined and offered birth control if she so desires.

Most women are ready to leave the hospital within a day or so after an uncomplicated vaginal delivery. The minimum time a woman needs before she could go home is about six to eight hours, but most women choose to stay a longer to rest and recover. If the woman agrees to a home visit in the first few days of delivery, she probably can go home safely without having to stay in the hospital longer than a few hours. First time moms should probably be seen a week after delivery as they may have more questions and more problems than moms who have had children before. They often require extra guidance regarding breastfeeding, since they have never done it before.

Women who have had a cesarean section tend to need to stay in the hospital for at least three days or more. Any woman who has had a postpartum hemorrhage should stay longer than a few hours and optimally stay at least twenty-four hours before they can be discharged.

One of the most important goals for a woman after giving birth is the establishment of adequate milk production from her breasts. Breastfeeding does not come easily to every woman and some women need the assistance of a breastfeeding counselor to acclimate her to the breastfeeding process. The breast milk does not fully come in for a couple of days after birth and the new mother should know this is normal and her baby will not starve if left to drink just the colostrum in the first few days after birth.

The postpartum woman should be told to refrain from sexual intercourse for the first three weeks after the birth of her child. This will allow any vaginal or perineal lacerations to heal and make the act of intercourse something pleasurable and not painful.

The postpartum woman also needs to have patient education around the presence of a fever and should report any fever greater than thirty-eight degrees Celsius to the doctor as there can be serious underlying problems that may manifest as a fever. The main causes of a puerperal fever include a urinary tract infection, a respiratory tract infection, mastitis, or a breast infection. Thrombophlebitis, either deep or superficial may present as a fever. Most urinary tract infections are secondary to streptococcus or Staphylococcus aureus, rather than Gram-negative organisms. Anaerobic bacteria also cause urinary tract infections in the puerperal woman.

Some women will have what is known as a secondary postpartum hemorrhage that occurs beyond the first postpartum day. It generally occurs between the fifth and fourteenth postpartum day and can be severe enough to result in hypotension and shock. It is not the type of bleeding that resolves spontaneously and usually requires medical intervention. The main cause for this type of bleeding is some sort of genital infection that may or may not be secondary to a retained placental fragment. In women who've had a cesarean section, the main cause of secondary postpartum bleeding is dehiscence and breakdown of the uterine incision. In rare cases, postpartum bleeding is secondary to a choriocarcinoma or a hydatidiform mole. Cases of bleeding that are associated with heavy bleeding usually mean the problem is secondary to an infectious source.

Postpartum Care at Home

Patient education should be given to all women as they leave the hospital or birthing center. She should understand that breast engorgement is normal and means that the breasts are preparing to make breast milk for the newborn. She needs to be taught how to care for her breasts to be able to provide sustenance for the infant without developing cracked nipples or mastitis. Some cases of mastitis are unavoidable but, if the mother keeps breastfeeding and takes antibiotics, these sorts of breast complications will soon abate.

New mothers should also understand that for various reasons, constipation is normal after a vaginal or cesarean birth. Things like hemorrhoids that developed during childbirth and healing episiotomy scars will also contribute to painful defecation and constipation. Most women can do well by increasing fluid intake and taking in more fiber in the diet. Rarely are laxatives be necessary in the postpartum period.

The episiotomy will need special care after a vaginal delivery. Many women do well with Sitz baths at home and using a squirt bottle to wash off the perineum after voiding or a bowel movement. Education around caring for the episiotomy and reassurance that things like painful sitting and painful bowel movements are normal and will soon abate as the stitches heal and dissolve inside the wound.

Other things that may crop up in the postpartum state include hot flashes and cold flashes, which come from an abrupt change in hormonal environment. Urinary and fecal incontinence may happen after a particularly difficult vaginal delivery. Most women will experience uterine cramping in the days after the delivery as the uterus contracts. Breastfeeding moms tend to have more cramping when the infant is suckling because the act of suckling releases hormones that increase uterine contractions. The lochia will initially be very heavy and red in color but gradually will lighten in the amount of flow, with the color turning to yellow or white as it gradually fades away. Women will immediately weigh about twelve to thirteen pounds less than their last pregnancy weight. Additional weight will come off as the body sheds extra water weight and as the woman increases her physical activity after birth.

Postpartum Birth Control

It is possible to become pregnant even before the woman has her first period after giving birth. This is much less likely in a woman who is exclusively breastfeeding at least eight times per day and in women who don't get their period while breastfeeding. It is still possible to get pregnant while breastfeeding, particularly as the child is being weaned and begins to eat some solid foods. There are birth control options for breastfeeding mothers that include barrier methods, an IUD, and the mini-pill, which contains only progestins. Ideally, issues around birth control should be discussed prior to leaving the hospital after the birth but, if this isn't feasible, it should be discussed at the six-week postpartum visit.

Breastfeeding Issues

The breastfeeding new mother needs to be counseled in ways to take care of herself and her body as she carries on the important task of providing nutrition for her baby. She needs to eat a well-balanced, healthy diet that has enough calories to sustain her and her infant. She needs to have a high fluid intake throughout her breastfeeding time and should aim to have a glass of water every time her infant breastfeeds. Caffeinated beverages should be avoided as they can dehydrate the woman and can make the baby fussy and irritable.

The breastfeeding mother should ideally be given access to a lactation specialist, both for at home and while beginning the breastfeeding process in the hospital. She need to know how to relieve clogged milk ducts through the act of breast massage, frequent breastfeeding, and the use of a warm shower to unclog the blocked milk ducts. Warm compresses can also be applied to increase the circulation to the breasts and to unclog blocked ducts.

Anytime a breastfeeding woman develops a fever, there should be a high index of suspicion for mastitis, especially if there are obvious findings like a red and tender breast. Antibiotics are necessary for a breast infection and there will be no need to stop breastfeeding. In fact, breastfeeding will stimulate the blood flow to the breast and will improve the outlook of mastitis if the antibiotic choice is compatible with breastfeeding.

Postpartum Psychiatric Conditions

The baby blues, postpartum psychosis, and postpartum depression occur in all ages of women, in all parts of the world, and in all ethnicities. The incidence of the baby blues is about 80 percent of all women. Women who have had difficulties with the pregnancy or the birth and women who are prone to low mood have an increased likelihood of developing the baby blues.

Baby blues is defined as the transient experience of low mood and irritability starting shortly after birth and lasting for up to two weeks. The symptoms are not very severe and do not adversely affect the postpartum woman's activities of daily living or her care of the infant.

The baby blues can develop shortly after pregnancy as the hormone fluctuations happen immediately after delivery. The main symptoms include the following:

- Rapid changes in mood
- Anxiousness
- Periods of sadness and irritability
- Feelings of being overwhelmed about mothering
- Episodes of crying
- Poor concentration
- Difficulty with eating too much or too little
- Insomnia or frequent awakenings at night

These symptoms last for only about one to two weeks after delivery.

Postpartum depression is much more severe and pervasive than the baby blues. It involves having a low mood, irritability, sleep disturbances, and guilty feelings that occur after the delivery of an infant that last at least two weeks and interfere with activities of daily living and the ability of the woman to care for herself and her infant.

About 10 to 20 percent of women will have postpartum depression. Women who were depressed in pregnancy, have high stress levels, upheavals in life events, low incomes, decreased social support, the absence of a job, rigid parental beliefs, anxiety disorders, history of mental illness, and being a minority all increase the chance of developing postpartum depression.

The main symptoms of postpartum depression include the following:

- Low mood
- Periods of sadness
- Frequent episodes of crying
- Feeling insecure about being able to care for the infant
- Anxious symptoms related to caring for the infant
- Insomnia or frequent awakenings at night
- Eating too much or too little
- Having decreased ability to concentrate
- Having periods of confusion
- Being irritable
- Feeling isolated from others
- Feeling unwanted or worthless
- Feeling sensations of shame
- Feeling guilty about parenting skills
- Having increased anger outbursts
- Being unable to care for the infant because of symptoms

- Losing the ability to care for oneself because of symptoms
- A feeling of worthlessness
- Feelings of guilt, particularly around parenting
- Feeling suicidal or having frequent thoughts of death

These symptoms can occur at any time within the first year of childbirth and must last at least two weeks to have the diagnosis of postpartum depression.

Postpartum psychosis is fortunately much less common than the baby blues and postpartum depression. It is an extremely severe illness with the onset of symptoms happening usually within two weeks after delivery. The postpartum woman will experience psychotic symptoms, such as hallucinations, irritability, unusual thought patterns, mood swings, and difficulty sleeping that last for at least two weeks.

Postpartum psychosis occurs in 1-2 out of every one thousand pregnancies. Women at the greatest risk for this disorder are those with previous psychiatric illnesses or those who suffered from psychosis during pregnancy. The disorder usually begins with two weeks after giving birth.

Symptoms of postpartum psychosis include the following:

- Periods of paranoia
- Episodes of confusion
- Feelings of disorientation
- Being obsessed about caring for the infant
- Hallucinations, which are usually auditory in nature
- Insomnia or frequent awakenings at night
- Homicidal or violent thoughts related to the infant
- Suicidal thoughts or suicide attempts

Because the symptoms of postpartum psychosis are severe, it is considered a psychiatric emergency and almost always results in hospitalization for psychiatric treatment.

No one knows the exact etiology of the baby blues, postpartum depression, and postpartum psychosis. It is believed that both internal and external factors play a role in the development of postpartum psychiatric disorders. Abrupt decreases in progesterone and estrogen occur after pregnancy, which is believed to trigger emotional changes in susceptible women.

Women who have little social support, have a low socioeconomic status, a complicated birth, an unwanted gender of baby, are not working, have a history of mental illness, or experienced an anxiety, depressive, or psychotic disorder during pregnancy are at a greater risk of developing both postpartum depression. Women with postpartum psychosis are at an elevated risk of suicide.

Treatment of Postpartum Psychiatric Disorders

There is no special treatment necessary for the baby blues. The woman's symptoms tend to resolve spontaneously, and she will require only supportive measures such as reassurance and brief talk therapy. These interventions are only necessary if the woman feels she needs these things to support her in the few weeks that this emotional upheaval lasts.

Women with postpartum depression who aren't breastfeeding can easily be treated with selective serotonin reuptake inhibitors, such as fluoxetine, paroxetine, escitalopram, sertraline, and fluvoxamine. There are risks to taking these drugs in breastfeeding mothers, so the risks need to be weighed against the benefits before using these drugs. Some women, particularly those who don't want to take medications, will benefit from electroconvulsive therapy as this has no risks for the infant. Psychotherapy is also a first-line treatment for postpartum depression, with cognitive behavioral and family-centered therapies being the best options.

Women with postpartum psychosis represent a psychiatric emergency as these women are significantly symptomatic and are at an elevated risk of suicide and homicide. These women are often treated aggressively with atypical antipsychotic medications, such as ziprasidone, quetiapine, and risperidone. Other antipsychotics, such as olanzapine, haloperidol, and clozapine have been used and have been found to be effective in treating these patients. Psychotherapy generally only helps psychoses after the initial crisis has been averted. Family-centered therapy can then help the patient and her family pick up the pieces left behind as the patient recovers from this severe disorder. Electroconvulsive therapy can be used to decrease any depressive symptoms.

Key Takeaways

- The postpartum or puerperal state begins as soon as the placenta has delivered and arbitrarily ends at six weeks after birth, even though changes continue to happen after this arbitrary deadline.
- Breastfeeding mothers, particularly first-time mothers, will need extra support around the initiation and continuation of breastfeeding.
- The most common cause of a postpartum fever is a urinary tract infection, although other types of infections, including genital and uterine infections can play a role in getting a fever in the postpartum state.
- Birth control options should be addressed at the time of discharge from the hospital and reiterated during the six-week postpartum visit.
- Postpartum psychiatric disorders include the baby blues, postpartum depression, and postpartum psychosis.

Quiz

1. You are evaluating a new mother who is about to be discharged from the hospital after an uncomplicated vaginal delivery. What is the minimum amount of time the woman should be in the hospital before allowing her to go home?
    a. Three hours
    b. Six hours

c. Twelve hours
d. Forty-eight hours

Answer: b. Women should stay in the hospital or birthing center at least six hours after giving birth but can be discharged after that time if they are medically stable.

2. A woman presents to the emergency room with a red, tender breast and a fever. She is nursing a two-week-old infant. How should this presentation be managed?
   a. Restrict breastfeeding to the normal breast until the infection resolves.
   b. Instruct the woman to use hot compresses on the affected breast.
   c. Provide the woman with an antibiotic that does not penetrate breast milk.
   d. Provide the woman with an antibiotic that is safe when ingested by the newborn.

Answer: d. The woman who is breastfeeding and has mastitis should be allowed to continue breastfeeding on the affected breast and should be given an antibiotic that is safely ingested by newborns.

3. You are counseling a twenty-five-year-old woman who is nursing her two-month-old infant and wants something for birth control. What is the most effective birth control method you can prescribe or recommend for her?
   a. Diaphragm
   b. Male condom
   c. Mini-pill
   d. Estradiol/Progestin pill

Answer: c. The safest and most effective form of birth control for a nursing mother is the mini-pill, which contains only progestins and can be ingested by the breastfeeding infant.

4. You are caring for a thirty-year-old woman who is breastfeeding and has clinical signs and symptoms of postpartum depression. What treatment can be given safely to her while she breastfeeds?
   a. Nortriptyline
   b. Amitriptyline
   c. Fluoxetine
   d. Electroconvulsive therapy

Answer: d. A nursing mother can have antidepressants while nursing but there is a risk to the infant by doing so. For this reason, the safest option is to use electroconvulsive therapy, which does not harm the infant in any way.

5. You are managing the care of a postpartum woman. At what time can you expect her uterus to shrink to its pre-pregnancy size?
    a. Two weeks
    b. Four weeks
    c. Six weeks
    d. It will never shrink to the pre-pregnancy size

Answer: d. While the uterus will continue to shrink until six weeks' postpartum, it will never actually shrink to its pre-pregnancy size after a woman has given birth.

6. A woman you are evaluating in the clinic is one week postpartum and has symptoms of tearfulness and low mood that have not impacted her sleep, appetite, or her care of her newborn. How long can you tell the woman these symptoms are likely to last?
    a. Two weeks
    b. Six weeks
    c. Two months
    d. Six months

Answer: a. The woman has symptoms suggestive of the baby blues. These generally only last for two weeks after the birth of the child and spontaneously get better without treatment.

7. The husband of a postpartum woman calls to say his wife is hallucinating and has illogical thoughts. She is unable to care for her infant and he needs to do all the childcare. What advice should you give him?
    a. He should make an appointment for his wife to see a psychiatrist.
    b. He should start giving her an antipsychotic drug that you will provide for her.
    c. He needs to have her seen urgently in the emergency department.
    d. He needs to pick up a prescription for an antidepressant medication to give her.

Answer: c. The woman with these symptoms likely has postpartum psychosis, which is a psychiatric emergency requiring urgent medical attention. She needs to be seen in the emergency department and probably admitted to an inpatient psychiatric unit.

8. You are discussing postpartum depression with a woman who is having the symptoms of the disorder. What do you tell her the incidence is of this problem among postpartum women?
    a. One to two percent
    b. Four to six percent
    c. Ten to twenty percent
    d. Twenty to thirty percent

Answer: c. The incidence of postpartum depression among women who have just given birth is about ten to twenty percent, so it needs to be screened for in every woman who has recently given birth.

9. You are planning to discuss birth control methods and contraception with your postpartum patients. At what point after childbirth should you discuss this with your patients?
    a. At the time of hospital discharge
    b. At two weeks' postpartum
    c. At the six-week postpartum visit
    d. By the sixth postpartum month

Answer: a. As a woman can get pregnant before her six-week postpartum visit, a discussion of birth control options should occur before her discharge from the hospital. Any time after that may be too late for adequate contraception to be in place.

10. A one-week postpartum mother presents to the clinic with the complaint of constipation after having an unremarkable vaginal delivery without an episiotomy. What can you recommend for her or prescribe her that will help this problem?
    a. Bisacodyl suppositories
    b. Fluids and increased fiber
    c. Milk of Magnesia
    d. Mylanta

Answer: b. In general, nothing is required for the treatment of constipation after giving birth apart from increasing fluids and adding fiber to the diet.

Chapter 7: Medical Conditions in Pregnancy

While most women begin and end their pregnancy in good health, some have pre-existing medical problems that may adversely affect the pregnancy. They may also develop medical problems during pregnancy that are unrelated to the pregnancy but require medical attention from the obstetrician or by a specialist.

Hypertension and Pregnancy

One of the most common medical conditions seen in pregnancy is hypertension, which affects up to three percent of all pregnancies. According to the National High Blood Pressure Program Working Group on High Blood Pressure in Pregnancy, there are four types of hypertension seen in pregnancy. These include chronic hypertension, preeclampsia-eclampsia, preeclampsia superimposed on chronic hypertension, and gestational hypertension. Of these, only preeclampsia-eclampsia and preeclampsia superimposed on chronic hypertension are considered dangerous, as they may lead to maternal seizures and pregnancy complications.

Recently, the American College of Obstetricians and Gynecologists Committee on Obstetric Practice provided updated guidelines as to the expected management of women who present in pregnancy with the acute onset of severe hypertension. According to their guidelines, any acute onset, severe hypertension that can be accurately measured using a sphygmomanometer lasting longer than fifteen minutes in pregnancy should be considered an emergency medical situation. The treatment for this, should it happen in pregnancy, is to provide either intravenous labetalol or intravenous hydralazine as first line agents. These same medications should be used in postpartum women, who may also receive oral nifedipine to stabilize the blood pressure. Pregnant women who have asthma, coronary artery disease, or congestive heart failure should only receive hydralazine, as labetalol can worsen their medical condition.

When the need for urgent treatment arises and an intravenous line cannot be established, oral nifedipine should be given while access to an intravenous site can be achieved. An alternative is to give two hundred milligrams of labetalol through orally. Labetalol can be repeated in thirty minutes if there isn't an adequate response after the first dose.

While magnesium sulfate is often used in the treatment of preeclampsia/eclampsia, it is not an antihypertensive medication, rather used to prevent seizures in patients with severe preeclampsia and to control active seizures in eclampsia. Sodium nitroprusside is the treatment of choice in non-pregnant women with severe hypertension but is not recommended in pregnancy unless the hypertension is life-threatening and refractory. Sodium nitroprusside carries a risk of cyanide and thiocyanide toxicity in both the mother and fetus, and there is a risk of increased intracranial pressure and cerebral edema when given to pregnant women.

Some pregnant women have preexisting hypertension, known as chronic hypertension. The definition of this is the finding of elevated blood pressure at any time prior to the pregnancy or prior to the twentieth week of pregnancy. When hypertension is first identified in pregnancy and when the woman is less than twenty weeks' gestation at the time, these blood pressure elevations are rarely secondary to the pregnancy and usually mean she has chronic hypertension.

On the other hand, if there are elevations in the pregnant woman's blood pressure after twenty weeks' gestation, this is probably secondary to the pregnancy and is deemed gestational hypertension or preeclampsia. The finding of protein in the urine clinches the diagnosis of preeclampsia as opposed to gestational hypertension or chronic hypertension. Preeclampsia affects up to five percent of all pregnancies and ten percent of first-time pregnancies. Up to twenty-five percent of pregnancies in which the woman had preexisting hypertension, preeclampsia can complicate the pregnancy. Hypertension of any sort in pregnancy can be dangerous, resulting in maternal and fetal mortality and morbidity.

As mentioned, some pregnant women have chronic hypertension. Chronic hypertension is usually a primary disorder in up to ninety-five percent of cases and may be either essential hypertension (ninety percent of the time) or secondary to some other pathology (five percent of the time).

The major underlying disorders that can cause hypertension in women of childbearing years include polycystic kidney disease, glomerular kidney disease, interstitial disease of the kidneys, renal vascular disease (such as renal artery stenosis or fibromuscular dysplasia), excesses of mineralocorticoids, pheochromocytoma, elevated or low thyroid states, excesses of growth hormone, coarctation of the aorta, hyperparathyroidism, or the use of oral birth control pills. Preexisting hypertension has a high chance of leading to preeclampsia in pregnancy.

Chronic hypertension can be found in up to twenty-two percent of women of childbearing age, with varying prevalence, depending on the woman's ethnic background, age, and body mass index, with overweight women having a higher chance of having hypertension at a young age when compared to thinner women. About one percent of all pregnancies are adversely affected by the baseline diagnosis of chronic hypertension, with about six percent affected by gestational hypertension, and one to two percent affected by preeclampsia.

Treatment of Hypertension in Pregnancy

Pregnant women with significant hypertension during pregnancy need to be placed on bed rest, modified bed rest, or limit their physical activity, even though there isn't any proof that it lowers infant or maternal morbidity and mortality. Women with hypertension and the other clinical findings suggestive of preeclampsia need to be hospitalized and observed, with treatment focused on bringing down the blood pressure and avoiding seizure activity. Some women can be monitored at home if they are stable and compliant with treatment.

While the main risk in having chronic hypertension in pregnancy is the secondary finding of superimposed preeclampsia, there is no evidence to suggest that medical treatment of mildly elevated blood pressure readings will reduce the incidence of secondary preeclampsia. In a normal pregnancy, a woman's average blood pressure drops ten to fifteen millimeters Hg during the first half of the pregnancy.

Women with mild chronic hypertension before getting pregnant in the range of one hundred forty and one hundred sixty systolic, have a similar decline in blood pressure so that they may be able to be taken off their antihypertensive medications during the pregnancy. Diastolic pressures of greater than one hundred ten millimeters Hg are considered significantly high and carry an elevated risk of intrauterine growth restriction, placental abruption, and seizures. Systolic blood pressure readings higher than one hundred sixty systolic will place the woman at risk for the development of an intracerebral hemorrhage. This means that any pregnant woman with a blood pressure that is higher than one hundred sixty systolic and one hundred ten diastolic should be actively managed with antihypertensive drugs.

The main goal of the pharmacological management of hypertension in pregnancy is to keep the blood pressure below 160/100, although lower blood pressure readings are preferable. Women with longstanding hypertension and preexisting end-organ damage should be placed on antihypertensive medications at much lower blood pressure readings as they already have hypertensive complications.

Any pregnant woman who presents with a blood pressure reading of 160/110 or higher at any point in the pregnancy requires admission to the hospital and rapid reduction of her blood pressure. If there is protein in the urine suggestive of preeclampsia, anticonvulsant therapy should be administered along with the antihypertensive agent. The most effective preventative against preeclampsia-connected seizures is magnesium sulfate, although phenytoin can be used with less efficacy.

Treating hypertension in pregnancy and in the postpartum state usually means the infant is getting some of the drugs used to treat the problem in utero or through breast milk. Because the US Food and Drug Administration have categorized pregnancy drugs in categories such as A, B, C, D, and X, these guidelines can be used to make recommendations as to the type of antihypertensive drug to use. There are some antihypertensive agents that aren't as highly excreted in breast milk, making them attractive options. The first line agents for the management of pregnancy-related hypertension and chronic hypertension in pregnancy are methyldopa and labetalol. Methyldopa has a good safety record but isn't very effective in severe hypertension. Labetalol, on the other hand, works quickly when given intravenously and can be used for severe hypertension. The only real risk of this medication in pregnancy is that it can cause transient neonatal hypoglycemia after birth so the infant should be monitored for this side effect.

Some of the relationship between labetalol and neonatal hypoglycemia is limited by the higher than average chance that a hypotensive woman will also have gestational diabetes or preexisting diabetes. Thus, the etiology behind this hypoglycemic response in neonates of hypertensive mothers on labetalol is likely multifactorial.

Long acting Nifedipine is a reasonable medication that can treat chronic hypertension in postpartum women. Shorter acting drugs can be used if the woman has a heart condition, such as nadolol and metoprolol. The only antihypertensive drugs not recommended in pregnancy are ACE inhibitors and angiotensin II receptor blockers.

ACE inhibitors should not be given in pregnancy as they can cause fetal renal dysgenesis, which can lead to fetal demise in the second and third trimesters. There is also an increased risk of heart malformations and malformations of the central nervous system in the fetus if this class of drugs is used in the first trimester. Some of the birth defects may be due to the extreme degree of hypertension seen in some newly pregnant women.

While obstetricians and medical doctors care for hypertensive pregnant women all the time, complicated cases may need expertise beyond that which can be provided by these specialists. In severe or refractory cases, a perinatologist may need to become involved to manage both the mother's experiences and complications of hypertension as well as the possible fetal outcomes that may occur with untreated chronic hypertension and the treatment of the condition.

Of note, women with mild chronic hypertension often don't require any antihypertensive therapy during pregnancy as there will be a natural drop in blood pressure that will often be in the normal range. The use of antihypertensive agents in pregnancy to bring the blood pressure down does not decrease a woman's chances of having preeclampsia later in the pregnancy and increases the risk of intrauterine growth restriction. Treatment is always recommended, however, for sustained blood pressure readings of more than 160/100.

Preeclampsia

Women with mild, already-diagnosed preeclampsia far from their due date or who have labile blood pressure readings secondary to gestational hypertension or chronic hypertension should be hospitalized, closely watched, and treated for both their hypertension and the prevention of a seizure, as can be seen in preeclampsia and eclampsia. Frequent fetal monitoring should take place while the woman is hospitalized and bed rest should be reinforced. Blood work is periodically done if the patient's health is poor and the overriding priority is to get the fetus out of the mother's uterus as soon as it is feasibly possible.

While in the hospital, the woman should have daily evaluations that include a fundoscopic exam, looking for retinal edema or retinal spasm. The lungs should be evaluated for evidence of fluid overload. The heart should be monitored for arrhythmias or abnormal heart sounds. The abdomen should be evaluated for tenderness of the liver. The extremities should be evaluated for peripheral edema and a neurological examination should be done to evaluate the woman for clonus, which can indicate preeclampsia. The patient should also be at a facility where a preterm birth can be managed should it be necessary to induce the woman early because of severe hypertension and fetal distress.

While the woman remains pregnant with hypertension, a fetal evaluation should be done at least two times per week, using things like non-stress testing and biophysical profile evaluations supervised by the obstetrician. If there is evidence of deterioration of the fetal status, an imminent delivery should occur by whatever means seems safest and most feasible.

It should be noted that, even though there are antihypertensive agents to bring down the blood pressure in preeclampsia, it doesn't mean that the disease progression has stopped so there needs to be ongoing evaluation and management for seizures and other effects seen in preeclampsia.

Women who have preeclampsia that required hospitalization require follow-up after they are discharged home. This is to ensure that the blood pressure remains normalized and that the lab work isn't serious. An obstetric internist, obstetrician, or a family physician can provide this follow up care.

It is important to remember that delivery of the child doesn't necessarily cure the preeclampsia right away and the symptoms may worsen after the delivery. Some women may develop preeclampsia after the delivery even if they had normal blood pressures in pregnancy. Any blood pressure reading of

160/110 mm Hg or more should be emergently managed with parenteral antihypertensive medications. Oral medications may be given if the blood pressure is around 155/105. As the vasospasm causing this problem improves, the woman can be weaned off her medication.

The blood pressure elevations secondary to preeclampsia usually get better in the days to weeks following the birth but have been known to last up to three months. Any elevation in blood pressure beyond this is probably chronic hypertension.

Lab testing in preeclampsia should include a urine sample for proteinuria, blood work for thrombocytopenia, and liver enzymes to rule out HELLP syndrome in pregnancy. If the blood work does not normalize after the blood pressure returns to an acceptable state, further workup needs to be undertaken to rule out some other pathological condition.

Having preeclampsia and eclampsia puts the pregnant woman at risk for developing heart disease and atherosclerosis. They need ongoing evaluation for cardiac risk factors that include glucose tolerance testing, smoking cessation advice, cholesterol and triglyceride measurements, and obesity management. Any of these risk factors, if present, should be promptly addressed, particularly as the woman ages.

Diabetes and Pregnancy

There are three main types of diabetes. The first is type 1 diabetes, which is an autoimmune diabetic state in which the individual makes antibodies against the Islets of Langerhans cells of the pancreas so that the pancreas makes no insulin. The second is type 2 diabetes, which is mostly a problem of insulin resistance. For much of the disease period, the pancreas puts out more insulin than normal but the cells are insulin-resistant so there is no usage of glucose as fuel. The third is gestational diabetes, which is an extension of type 2 diabetes but occurs only in pregnant women because of their increased insulin resistance.

Women who have diabetes before becoming pregnant either have no insulin or insulin resistance. This leads to high blood sugars and to the secondary problems associated with having diabetes while pregnant. The more severe the diabetes, the increased risk of prenatal, intrapartum, and postnatal complications.

As mentioned, diabetes in pregnancy can be gestational or pregestational. Either pregestational or gestational diabetes can be insulin-dependent, although, if a woman develops severe gestational diabetes, insulin is the only medication recommended for its management. Even type 2 diabetics must go on insulin therapy once they become pregnant.

Gestational diabetes is a medical condition involving elevated blood sugars that are above the acceptable range. It can be screened for by giving the woman a fifty-gram load of glucose in a syrupy solution and measuring the blood sugar reading after one hour. This is generally done on every pregnant woman at twenty-four weeks' gestation and sooner in women who are high risk because of sugar in the urine on exam or a strong family history of diabetes. A level of less than one hundred forty milligrams per deciliter is normal. Any number above that should be further evaluated and managed throughout the rest of pregnancy. These women have a greater than average chance of having type 2 diabetes later in life, particularly if they are obese. The problem is not a lack of insulin but rather an incidence of insulin resistance.

Women in pregnancy have a higher incidence of insulin resistance because there are hormones produced by the placenta that naturally antagonize insulin or that raise glucocorticoid levels that cause insulin resistance. This problem usually manifests itself at between twenty and twenty-four weeks' gestation. If the hormonal influences of the placenta overpower the insulin output of the pancreas, the blood sugar naturally rises.

Any woman can develop gestational diabetes but those at greatest risk includes women who have had a family history of diabetes, women who are obese, women with a previous stillbirth, a woman with a previous large infant, a history of birth defects in previous pregnancies, and being older than twenty-five years of age.

The main treatment for diabetes in pregnancy is lifestyle and dietary changes. Rarely are oral medications used to treat gestational diabetes and, if medication is necessary, insulin is usually prescribed for use during the pregnancy. The goal is to keep the blood sugars in good control to prevent the secondary complications that go along with having high blood sugars in pregnancy.

Infant complications can occur in unchecked gestational diabetes. There can be birth defects if the blood sugar is elevated in the first trimester. However, women with pure gestational diabetes generally don't have blood sugar elevations until the second or third trimester. After birth in pregnancies complicated by gestational diabetes, there can be several infant complications.

The first and most common effect to the infant is macrosomia, which means the infant is larger than normal for their gestational age. The woman's blood has an elevated glucose level and this molecule crosses the placental barrier, causing the fetus to put out more insulin and store excess glucose in the blood stream as fat. This leads to the finding of macrosomia, which contributes to a greater chance of a birth injury.

Hypoglycemia is another postpartum neonatal complication. It happens in the first few hours after the birth of the baby. The baby is suddenly in an environment where there isn't a steady supply of glucose. The baby's insulin levels are still high, which results in a sudden drop of blood sugar that can last for several hours and can be life-threatening. The baby born to a gestational diabetic mother needs early blood sugar monitoring after birth, early feeding, and possibly parenteral glucose.

Too much glucose or too much insulin in the baby's blood can cause maturational delay of the lungs with respiratory difficulty shortly after birth, especially if the infant is born prior to thirty-seven weeks' gestation.

Infectious Diseases and Pregnancy

Infections can occur during pregnancy that can harm or kill the fetus. Even ordinary infections in pregnancy, such as urinary tract infections, can cause fever and uterine irritability that requires treatment to avoid preterm labor and a preterm birth. Rarely, a urinary tract infection can spread to the uterus and can cause chorioamnionitis or an infection of the membranes around the fetus.

Toxoplasmosis is a very dangerous infection in pregnancy. Toxoplasmosis is a parasitic infection from an organism known as Toxoplasma gondii. While many people can have toxoplasmosis without any symptoms, individuals with a poor immune system will have more serious disease. Babies who get toxoplasmosis in utero will have an increased chance of being born with birth defects and serious developmental delay. In pregnant women, the infection with toxoplasmosis can be extremely vague. The main symptoms are swollen lymph nodes, malaise, muscle aches, joint pain, and flu-like symptoms that can last as few as a couple of days or several weeks. Mothers can be checked for the antibody to toxoplasmosis. If she develops the disease, an ultrasound, amniocentesis, and cord blood evaluations should be performed to see if the fetus is affected.

The treatment for toxoplasmosis is to administer antibiotics as soon as it is determined the woman is infected. Prevention is key, which involves using gloves during gardening as cats often carry the toxoplasmosis parasite in their feces and commonly defecate outdoors. Soap and water should be used after working outdoors and prior to the preparation of food. Pregnant woman should avoid changing a cats litterbox, and when necessary, should use gloves when cleaning the litter box. Litter box cleaning should also take place daily, before the toxoplasmosis has a chance to grow in the stool. Pregnant women should also avoid handling raw, and all cutting boards, knives, and other utensils exposed to raw meat, should be carefully washed with soap and water. All meat should be cooked until it is well done.

Food Poisoning

Pregnant women with food poisoning can suffer from dehydration, which can adversely affect her pregnancy. Food poisoning can come from viruses, such as enterovirus, bacteria, like Shigella, Campylobacter, and Clostridium, and parasites. While some only affect the gastrointestinal tract, others can spread to the fetus in utero and can cause meningitis, pneumonia, and sudden death in fetuses and newborns. To prevent this complication, all meat products should be thoroughly cooked, all vegetables should be washed prior to eating, and pregnant woman shouldn't eat or work with raw foods. Women who are pregnant should also avoid unpasteurized milk. Handwashing and the washing of utensils is vital if a pregnant woman must work with raw foods.

Sexually Transmitted Diseases

Pregnant women are not immune to getting sexually transmitted diseases and some of these diseases can adversely affect the pregnancy. The main STDs to worry about include Chlamydia, hepatitis B, herpes, HIV, syphilis, and gonorrhea.

Contracting chlamydia during pregnancy can increase the risk of the pregnancy ending in a miscarriage, a premature birth, or a stillbirth. Women often have no symptoms with chlamydia but can have lower pelvic pain and an increase in vaginal discharge. If chlamydia is suspected, it can be cultured out of the cervical or vaginal discharge. If it is positive, the main treatment includes avoiding sexual intercourse until the woman and her sexual partner(s) have both been treated with azithromycin, erythromycin, or amoxicillin.

Hepatitis B is transmitted through the exchange of blood and bodily fluids from an infected person. While there are five different types of hepatitis, the ones to be concerned about in pregnancy include hepatitis B and hepatitis C. Hepatitis B is passed from mother to child at the time of birth when blood is exchanged. For this reason, all newborns receive the hepatitis B vaccination within a couple of weeks of birth. About ten percent of hepatitis B patients will have chronic disease and some of these will develop cirrhosis and liver cancer later in life. The virus can also be transmitted during the pregnancy.

The later in pregnancy a woman develops hepatitis B, the greater is her likelihood of passing the virus onto her infant. The typical signs that a woman has hepatitis B include malaise, nausea and vomiting, fatigue, abdominal pain, anorexia, and jaundice (although the infection can develop without obvious symptoms. Women are routinely checked for hepatitis B at the first prenatal visit so that if they have the disease, they can receive hepatitis B immune globulin. Infants born to woman who are positive for hepatitis B will receive hepatitis B immune globulin along with the hepatitis B vaccine in the first twelve hours of life. Even babies unexposed to hepatitis B will get the vaccination. Preterm babies of Hep B negative mothers can be immunized a month after birth, with the full vaccination series to be completed in infancy.

Women with HIV disease pose a special problem in pregnancy. She will have a twenty-five percent chance of giving the virus to her fetus in utero or at the time of birth. HIV impairs the mother's immune system and puts her at risk for infections and cancer during her pregnancy. As HIV can be passed through breast milk, mothers who are HIV positive should not nurse their infants. Women are given antiretroviral therapy during pregnancy to diminish transmission of the virus and babies born to HIV mothers are given a short course of antiretroviral therapy after birth as prophylaxis against possible viral exposure during birth.

Because an HIV infection can be prevented in neonates, all pregnant women are screened for HIV at the time of the first prenatal visit. When detected, mothers receive treatment to prevent transmission of the virus during pregnancy and to keep the mother as healthy as possible during pregnancy.

Herpes is a sexually transmitted disease that leads to genital vesicles that burn and itch, open, and spread the virus to the person's sexual partners. Herpes can also spread to the infant under certain circumstances. While the membranes are intact, which is the bulk of pregnancy, there is no risk to the fetus, but the infant can develop herpes at the time of birth if the mother has an active infection during a vaginal delivery. Women should practice safe sex during pregnancy because having a primary herpes infection during pregnancy increases the chances of passing the disease onto the infant. Women in pregnancy can be given an antiviral medication like acyclovir or valaciclovir both during pregnancy and around the time of birth to suppress any active lesions, allowing for a safe vaginal delivery without the chance of transmitting the virus to the infant in childbirth.

All pregnant women are screened for the presence of syphilis with a rapid plasma reagin test at the time of the first prenatal visit. This is because a woman who is pregnant can pass the infection on to her baby in utero as the pathogen can cross the placenta from the woman's bloodstream at any time in the pregnancy or delivery. Syphilis that is treated in pregnancy will not generally affect the baby, but untreated syphilis can result in a fifty percent chance of infecting the fetus. Treated women can still pass on the infection but the risk is only about one to two percent. Babies affected by syphilis can die as part of a miscarriage, a near-term stillbirth, or can die after being born. Babies who live can have serious neurological impairments. Preterm births and intrauterine growth restriction are relatively common complications of untreated syphilis in pregnant women.

Gonorrhea can affect pregnant woman with adverse outcomes in the pregnancy. The mother may have an increased chance of a first trimester miscarriage, an increased chance of gonorrheal chorioamnionitis, premature rupture of the membranes, and premature birth of her infant. These things tend to occur primarily in untreated women, so it is imperative that women with symptoms of gonorrhea or a known gonorrhea exposure get treated while she is pregnant and before having a vaginal birth. If the woman has untreated gonorrhea and has a vaginal birth, the infection can enter the eyes of the fetus, resulting in a severe eye infection. Most states mandate the use of eyedrops to be given to all newborns immediately after birth even though the gonorrhea status of the mother isn't known. Known gonorrhea cases at the time of childbirth are treated by giving both the mother and the newborn oral systemic antibiotics. Untreated babies can become blind, can have septicemia, and can have gonorrheal meningitis.

Medications and Pregnancy

Whenever a woman is pregnant, she may need medications and may wonder whether she should use the medications during her pregnancy. Because medications can cross the placental barrier, the pregnant woman should discuss taking medications with her doctor before using anything, even if it is over-the-counter. Most of the time, things like acetaminophen are safe in pregnancy but it is a good idea to ask the pharmacist or doctor before taking any medication.

Some women must, by necessity, take prescription medications for chronic health problems they had before becoming pregnant. A woman anticipating a pregnancy should see her doctor before she gets pregnant to initiate appropriate medication management for when she becomes pregnant. Women already pregnant should see the obstetrician or their family doctor to see which medication changes can be made before having to take medications for too long during pregnancy. It should be noted that most of the adverse effects of medications will be most harmful during the first trimester. Thus, once the woman learns she is pregnant, the medication she takes may already have had an adverse effect on her fetus.

The US Food and Drug Administration has created a letter system that helps doctors, pharmacists, and patients understand which medications are the safest to take during pregnancy. The letter system is based on animal testing, human testing, and what is known about the effects of a particular medication on a pregnant woman. For example, medications in Category A have been tested in pregnant women and have been found to be completely safe for use in pregnancy. Category B medications are those that have been found to be safe for humans, but no pregnancy testing has been done. Pregnancy Category C means the drug hasn't been tested enough to say whether the drug is safe in pregnancy. Pregnancy Category D medications have been tested and have some adverse effects in humans. Pregnancy Category X medications have been found to be dangerous for use in pregnant woman and should never be used in pregnancy. The drugs thalidomide, benzodiazepines, Accutane, and many birth control medications are considered Category X medications.

Key Takeaways

- The most common health concern in pregnant women is hypertension, which can predate the pregnancy or a complication of the pregnancy.
- There are innate problems with insulin resistance in pregnancy so that pregnant women have a higher than normal risk of diabetes while pregnant. This type of diabetes is known as gestational diabetes.
- Infants born to diabetic mothers can have several health problems, including macrosomia and neonatal hypoglycemia.
- Several infectious diseases can affect a pregnant woman, some of which only affect the mother, while others can be passed from mother to fetus through the blood or from ascending into the uterus from the birth canal.

Quiz

1. The woman is in her third trimester and found to have a resting blood pressure of 165/100. What is the next test that should be done to evaluate this finding?
    a. Electrocardiogram
    b. Brachial ankle index
    c. Urine dipstick for protein
    d. Serum protein level

Answer: c. What isn't known is whether this patient's hypertension is essential hypertension, gestational hypertension, or preeclampsia. The test that can help define this is a urine dipstick for protein, which will show protein in the urine in cases of preeclampsia.

2. The woman being evaluated in the emergency department is 32-weeks' gestational age with a blood pressure reading of 155/95. The urinalysis shows 3+ protein in the urine. What can be given to her to prevent eclampsia?
    a. IV nitroprusside
    b. Oral labetalol
    c. IV hydralazine
    d. IV magnesium sulfate

Answer: d. While antihypertensive medications can easily bring the blood pressure down, they don't prevent the seizures associated with eclampsia. Only IV magnesium sulfate can do this.

3. The patient is a 32-year-old multiparous woman with preeclampsia. At what point can she be safely assured of having no neurological complication from this problem?
    a. As soon as her blood pressure reaches below the 140/90 threshold
    b. As soon as she delivers her infant
    c. About three to four days after delivery
    d. After receiving at least forty-eight hours of labetalol orally

Answer: c. The woman's chance of seizures will diminish when she delivers but she is still at risk until about three to four days after the delivery.

4. The woman is having routine prenatal care for her first pregnancy. As part of this care, when should she have a one-hour glucose tolerance test for gestational diabetes?
   a. First prenatal visit
   b. Twelve weeks' gestational age
   c. Eighteen weeks' gestational age
   d. Twenty-four weeks' gestational age

Answer: d. A woman should receive a one-hour glucose tolerance test for gestational diabetes at twenty-four weeks' gestational age unless there is evidence that she has the disorder earlier in the pregnancy by history or lab findings.

5. A woman with type 2 diabetes on metformin becomes pregnant and sees her obstetrician. How will her diabetes be managed?
   a. She will remain on metformin but will monitor her blood sugars three times a day.
   b. She will stop the metformin and start a program of insulin therapy.
   c. She will stop the metformin and will begin a strict diet and exercise program for her diabetes.
   d. She will check blood sugars four times daily and will switch to Victoza (liraglutide)

Answer: b. Pregnant women with any type of diabetes need to be on insulin therapy for the duration of their pregnancy as oral drugs for diabetes are not considered as safe to be used in pregnant women.

6. A 35-year-old obese female is newly pregnant and has a baseline history of hypertension. What would be a first line medication to manage her hypertension?
   a. Labetalol
   b. Nifedipine
   c. Captopril
   d. Losartan

Answer: a. Labetalol is considered a first line agent for the management of hypertension in pregnancy. Nifedipine can be used for postpartum hypertension. Captopril and Losartan are contraindicated in pregnancy and should not be used.

7. An infant is born to a mother who is known to have chronic hepatitis B. How is this handled?
   a. The infant is given the hepatitis B vaccine at two weeks of age.
   b. The infant is tested for the virus and, if negative, is given the hepatitis B vaccine.
   c. The infant is given the hepatitis B immune globulin.
   d. The infant is given the hepatitis B immune globulin and the hepatitis B vaccine on the day of birth.

Answer: d. Any infant born to a mother known to have chronic hepatitis B should receive the hepatitis B immune globulin at the time of birth and should be vaccinated against hepatitis B within 12 hours of birth.

8. An infant is born to a mother who has an active gonorrhea infection at the time of a vaginal birth. How is the infant treated?
   a. The infant is given oral systemic antibiotics against gonorrhea.
   b. A blood culture is obtained, and the infant is treated if positive for gonorrhea.

    c. The infant is given erythromycin eye drops to protect against gonorrhea conjunctivitis.
    d. The infant is intravenous antibiotics against gonorrhea.

Answer: a. If an infant is born to a mother known to have vaginal or cervical gonorrhea, the infant and the mother should receive oral systemic coverage for the gonorrhea infection.

9. The pregnant woman is tested for HIV at the time of her first prenatal visit. For what reason is this done?
    a. Many pregnant women are high risk for HIV, so they should be screened whenever they become pregnant.
    b. There will be a lot of exchange of bodily fluids during the delivery, so the provider wants to know if there is a risk to the healthcare staff.
    c. The woman with HIV will be even more immunosuppressed during pregnancy so her status needs to be known.
    d. The woman with HIV disease can take antiretroviral agents during pregnancy to prevent maternal to fetal transmission in pregnancy.

Answer: d. The woman with HIV disease can take antiretroviral agents during pregnancy to prevent maternal to fetal transmission. Therefore, all pregnant women are screened for HIV, regardless of risk factors.

10. A woman has a rapid plasma reagin test at the time of her first prenatal visit. For what reason is this test done?
    a. This will determine if she will pass on syphilis to her newborn at the time of delivery.
    b. This offers an opportunity to treat syphilis before it can be passed to the fetus in utero.
    c. This will identify women who might have a preterm birth later in pregnancy.
    d. This will identify women who might develop tertiary syphilis during pregnancy.

Answer: b. Testing for syphilis with a rapid plasma reagin test will offer an opportunity for a woman to be treated for syphilis before the disease can be passed to the fetus in utero.

Chapter 8: Obstetrical Complications

Any pregnancy can come with complications, beginning from the first trimester, when ectopic pregnancies and spontaneous abortions can occur; to the second trimester, when things like placenta previa can occur; to the third trimester, when things like placental abruption and preeclampsia can occur. Some complications can be managed in an outpatient setting, while others are considered obstetrical emergencies that require urgent medical attention.

Amniotic Fluid Complications

The amniotic fluid surrounds the fetus during the time of gestation. It is necessary for the proper growth and development of the fetus. The two main complications of pregnancy include polyhydramnios, which is having too much amniotic fluid, and oligohydramnios, which is having too little amniotic fluid. Too much fluid can occur in cases of uncontrolled diabetes of pregnancy and in a multiple gestation pregnancy. Women with pregnancies complicated by birth defects in the fetus or Rh incompatibility will also have too much fluid. Too little amniotic fluid may be seen in certain fetal birth defects, in a stillbirth, or if the growth of the fetus is inadequate.

A normal amount of amniotic fluid protects the fetus from being injured, aids in the growth of the fetal lungs, and prevents infection from adversely affecting the fetus. The amount of fluid making up this space differs according to the gestational age with the most amniotic fluid present during thirty-six to thirty-seven weeks' gestation, when the fluid volume is between eight hundred and one thousand milliliters.

In the presence of polyhydramnios, up to twenty percent of newborns will be born with congenital birth defect. The obstetrician can evaluate the woman for polyhydramnios by doing an ultrasound and estimating the amount of fluid surrounding the fetus. An amniotic fluid index or AFI of more than twenty-four centimeters translates to the finding of a single pocket of fluid that is at least eight centimeters in depth and a total amniotic fluid volume of greater than two thousand milliliters. On the other hand, an AFI of less than seven centimeters indicates there is no fluid pocket on ultrasound that is more than two to three centimeters in depth.

The clinical picture of polyhydramnios will reveal a uterus that is large for gestational age. The most benign cause of this would be a multiple gestation pregnancy that can be easily identified by ultrasound. Fetal macrosomia, fetal hydrops with anasarca, duodenal atresia, tracheoesophageal fistula, fetal ascites, and fetal skeletal malformations may be associated with polyhydramnios. Children born with significant chromosomal abnormalities will also have an increased risk of polyhydramnios.

Oligohydramnios or too little amniotic fluid can be associated with an absence of the fetal kidneys or a fetal obstructive uropathy. Babies with Potter syndrome will have a flat face, kidney failure, hypertelorism, low set ears, and a lack of lung maturation from too little fluid in the amniotic sac. When these babies are born, they lack normal lung development and have an increased risk of death due to respiratory insufficiency at the time of birth. Other abnormalities that can be seen in oligohydramnios include a club foot, bowed legs, single umbilical artery, gastrointestinal atresia, and a narrowed chest cavity.

The first step in managing polyhydramnios is to prevent a preterm birth precipitated by overdistention of the uterus. The woman will need to be on bedrest and serial ultrasounds are necessary to follow the course of the problem. In cases of polyhydramnios secondary to fetal anemia, treatment includes giving an erythrocyte transfusion directly into the bloodstream or abdomen of the fetus in utero, which has the potential to prevent fetal congestive heart failure allowing pregnancy to proceed as long as possible.

The treatment of maternal oligohydramnios also involves bedrest with proper hydration, so the amniotic fluid will increase. Oral hydration of up to two liters per day will increase the AFI by thirty percent. Women who can't drink that much would benefit from intravenous hydration.

Placental Abruption

Placental abruption is also known as abruptio placentae. This condition is the premature separation of the placenta from the uterus, which can be life-threatening. Common associated complications include vaginal bleeding, an increase in uterine contractions, and acute fetal distress that comes from a lack of adequate fetal circulation. This condition is associated with significant maternal morbidity with the possibility of both maternal and fetal death.

The problem of placental abruption can come on because of maternal trauma, a maternal blood disorder, or from an unknown cause. There is hemorrhaging into the decidua basalis that separates the placenta from the inner uterine lining. When the bleeding escape from beneath the placenta, there will be obvious bright red vaginal bleeding. Sometimes the blood stays behind the placenta and the only finding is increased uterine cramping and fetal agitation from hypoxia.

The hematoma starts small and then enlarges over time, compressing normal blood vessels that are supposed to provide nutrients to the fetus. Sometimes the bleeding transverses the uterine wall and enters the peritoneal cavity. When this happens, it is called Couvelaire syndrome and can weaken the myometrium, leading to a rupture of the uterine wall, resulting in a serious obstetrical emergency.

A placental abruption can be diagnosed clinically but is aided by the ultrasound finding of a blood clot behind the placenta. A Kleinhauer-Betke test can be done, which is a test that looks for the presence of fetal blood cells in the mother's circulation. The abruption causes an untoward transfusion of fetal blood cells into the maternal bloodstream. The biggest problem with this is that it can cause Rh sensitization in Rh negative mother, which can be deadly to the Rh-positive fetus. Any placental abruption in an Rh-negative mother is an indication for Rhogam, which should neutralize any antibodies directed at the fetus from the Rh negative immune system in the mother.

The treatment of a placental abruption involves continuous fetal monitoring and insertion of least two large-bore intravenous catheters with crystalloid given to resuscitate the mother while blood is prepared for type and crossmatching. Blood should be given anytime the mother's circulatory status is unstable after receiving crystalloids. If the mother has a coagulopathy, this needs to be managed and Rh immune globulin should be provided for any mother that is known to be Rh-negative. Corticosteroids should be given intravenously in any preterm gestation as the likely outcome of the placental abruption is the urgent delivery of the fetus, regardless of the fetal age.

Ectopic Pregnancy

The basic definition of an ectopic pregnancy is any gestation that grows outside of the body of the uterus. The clear majority of ectopic pregnancies occur in the fallopian tubes but there can be ectopic pregnancies occurring in the cervical canal or even inside the abdominal cavity. The main cause of an ectopic pregnancy is the finding of scar tissue in the fallopian tube secondary to a past infection. Women who had a tubal ligation done prior to the age of thirty and have it reversed run a high risk of an ectopic pregnancy.

Ectopic pregnancies affect about one of fifty pregnancies. These are almost universally fatal to the fetus and can be fatal to the mother if left untreated. The longer an ectopic pregnancy can grow unchecked, the greater is the chance of rupture and sudden tubal hemorrhaging. About eighty percent of all ectopic pregnancies occur in the ampulla of the fallopian tube, while only one percent can be found in the peritoneal cavity.

The main symptoms seen in an ectopic pregnancy include amenorrhea from the presence of a pregnancy, abdominal or pelvic pain, and vaginal bleeding. Only about half of all women with an ectopic pregnancy will have these symptoms, making it difficult to diagnose. Many women will have secondary symptoms of pregnancy, such as nausea and breast engorgement so the index of suspicion that the pain is of an obstetrical origin is usually high.

The other symptoms that may point to the finding of an ectopic pregnancy include a fever, the sudden onset of weakness and dizziness, flu-like symptoms, vomiting, fainting spells, and even cardiac arrest with minimal warning. Signs that the problem represents a surgical emergency include the finding of abdominal rigidity, guarding of the abdomen, extreme abdominal tenderness, and evidence of hypovolemic shock. The uterus may be enlarged even in the absence of a gestation in the body of the organ and there may be cervical motion tenderness suggestive of an infection. If the ectopic pregnancy is large enough, a palpable adnexal mass will be noted, and bleeding will be present from shedding of the inner lining of the uterus.

The diagnosis can be made in several ways. A serial blood beta HCG level can be done with the expectation that a normal gestation will have doubling of the hormone level in forty-eight to seventy-two hours up to a maximum of about twenty thousand mIU per milliliter. Ectopic pregnancies will have lower HCG levels than expected and there will not be the expected doubling over the course of time. However, the HCG level must be higher than about one thousand five hundred mIU per milliliter to see a gestational sac in the uterus on transvaginal ultrasound in a healthy pregnancy. If the HCG is above this level and no gestational sac can be seen, there is the presumption then that an ectopic pregnancy exists somewhere other than the uterus.

If a gestational sac is seen in the uterus, even if there is no cardiac activity, the diagnosis of an ectopic pregnancy can usually be ruled out. However, it is technically possible to have an intrauterine pregnancy and an ectopic pregnancy at the same time. The transvaginal ultrasound is preferred because it can detect a gestational sac a week sooner than a trans-abdominal ultrasound. An empty uterus with an elevated HCG level should promote further evaluation as to the source of a probable ectopic pregnancy.

The gold standard for diagnosing an ectopic pregnancy is the laparoscopy examination. It is expensive and doesn't need to be done on every woman suspected of having an ectopic pregnancy. Besides that, it can miss up to four percent of ectopic pregnancies that are too early to cause a bulging of the fallopian tube. Nevertheless, patients in extreme pain and are hemodynamically unstable deserve to have an urgent laparoscopy that may also be used to remove the fallopian tube and its contents. Patients who have early ectopic pregnancies and no rupture of the fallopian tube can be treated medically with methotrexate, which will cause dissolution of the products of gestation. This might be enough to allow for normal tubal function in the future. In some cases, a stable patient can be monitored without treatment if there is HCG evidence of spontaneous dissolution of the pregnancy.

Methotrexate is an excellent medical treatment for early ectopic pregnancies, but cannot be used if the pregnancy is intrauterine, in immunosuppressed patients, or in patients who are severely anemic, leukopenic, or thrombocytopenia. Some women are sensitive to methotrexate and cannot receive the medication and women with active lung disease or peptic ulcer disease are not candidates for methotrexate. As methotrexate can be harmful to patients with significant liver or kidney disease, it is relatively contraindicated in these situations. Breastfeeding moms cannot receive methotrexate and it is contraindicated if the tube has already ruptured.

If surgery is required, the laparoscopic removal of the tube and its contents are preferable, but this may be impractical in cases of severe hemodynamic instability or in patients with ectopic pregnancies in the cornua of the uterus. In such cases, a full laparotomy is recommended to quickly enter the abdomen and maintain the patient's hemodynamic status while rapidly excising the bleeding products of conception that are no longer viable.

Miscarriage or Fetal Loss

A pregnancy that ends in miscarriage ends prior to twenty weeks' gestation although most end before twelve weeks' gestation. Any pregnancy loss after twenty weeks' gestation is called a fetal demise. About fifteen to twenty percent of all pregnancies end in miscarriage, with the most common etiology being a significant genetic defect or chromosomal abnormality. Fetal losses after twelve weeks' gestation and before twenty weeks' gestation are usually secondary to an incompetent cervix. This occurs when the cervix cannot hold the products of conception as they grow larger.

Many women believe that miscarriages happen because of falls, excessive exercise, sexual intercourse, stress, marital discord, or morning sickness. However, miscarriages occur as a defense mechanism in cases where the chance of fetal viability is nonexistent. Besides the most common cause of genetic defects, immune responses from the mother can cause a miscarriage. Unfortunately, even with extensive testing, some miscarriages have no definable etiology, which makes it difficult to make plans as to how to prevent another one from occurring.

Early miscarriages happen in the first trimester and make up about eighty percent of all miscarriages. Most occur much earlier than twelve weeks' gestation and a large proportion of them occur before the woman knows she is pregnant. There are a lot of intricate steps that begin with fertilization and end with successful implantation of the blastocyst. This means that, at any point in this process, things can go awry, leading to a miscarriage.

Late miscarriages are rare and happen in about one out of a thousand pregnancies. The woman usually knows she is pregnant and suffers a pregnancy loss between twelve weeks' and twenty weeks' gestation. The issues causing this type of miscarriage may be due to an incompetent cervix, an abnormal placenta, or a toxic exposure early in the pregnancy.

There are several types of miscarriage. For example, a chemical miscarriage happens when the egg was fertilized successfully but was never implanted. There will be a slight HCG rise resulting in a positive pregnancy test, but the ultrasound will fail to show any evidence of a pregnancy every being in the uterus. Bleeding happens only a few days after the expected menstrual period. A blighted ovum is another type of miscarriage. The egg is fertilized and implants so that a placenta develops. The placenta secretes HCG, yielding a positive pregnancy test but an ultrasound will show only an empty gestational sac.

A threatened miscarriage is a clinical term. It begins with heavy vaginal bleeding and the strong suspicion that a miscarriage is going to happen. If the products of conception remain in the uterus, the miscarriage is said to be "threatened" because it hasn't happened yet. There may even be the ultrasound or clinical finding of a heartbeat. About half of all threatened miscarriages progress no further and become healthy pregnancies. For this reason, many doctors will recommend bed rest for threatened miscarriages until they declare themselves as normal pregnancies or inevitable miscarriages.

An inevitable miscarriage involves heavy bleeding and an open cervix. The cervix is opening, indicating that whatever contents are in the uterus are likely to be expelled. These rarely go on to be normal pregnancies and it becomes a waiting game to see if the contents of the uterus will expel completely or if intervention to remove the products of conception will be necessary. A missed miscarriage involves a pregnancy loss without the typical bleeding and cramping. The only way to diagnose these is to have an ultrasound or the clinical evaluation that fails to reveal a fetal heartbeat at the expected time.

Most of the time, a miscarriage will have associated symptoms. The woman will experiance lower back pain or crampy pelvic pain associated with bleeding, the passage of clots, and the eventual passage of the products of conception. After the products of conception are expelled, the bleeding abates somewhat and goes away after about three days. Any signs of pregnancy the woman had will go away in the ensuing few days. Light spotting, does not portend a miscarriage and is normal in many healthy pregnancies, even though the finding can be unnerving for the newly pregnant mother.

Miscarriages can be diagnosed by doing serial HCG levels, which will fail to be high enough for a normal pregnancy or will fail to double over an expected period. An open cervix is highly indicative of an impending miscarriage. An ultrasound in the first trimester can often tell the difference between a healthy pregnancy and an inevitable miscarriage, but may be difficult in the very early stages of pregnancy. Sometimes even heavy bleeding will stop and a follow up ultrasound in a week or so will show the presence of a normal gestation.

If the patient experiences a relatively painless miscarriage, especially in the second trimester, the diagnosis of an incompetent cervix should be entertained. The treatment for an incompetent cervix before the pregnancy is lost is to place a cervical cerclage that closes the cervix helping retain the pregnancy until term or near term.

It can take up to two weeks for a miscarriage to progress normally and for all the retained placental fragments and embryonic tissue to be expelled. If it doesn't expel spontaneously, the doctor may need to perform a dilatation and curettage by opening the cervix and scraping out the products of conception to allow the uterus to heal, the resumption of normal periods, and the chance for a subsequent pregnancy to be healthy in the future. After successful evacuation of the uterus, the uterus is vulnerable to infection for up to two weeks so intercourse or the use of tampons is discouraged.

Even though miscarriages can happen to anyone, there are risk factors to keep in mind. Research has shown that women who are older at the time of conception have a higher risk for miscarriage as it is believed their eggs and the genetic makeup of their partner's sperm have more defects in them. In fact, one in three pregnancies among woman over the age of forty end in a miscarriage. Women who are deficient in vitamin D have a higher risk of miscarriage. Having too much vitamin A, on the other hand, seems to increase the risk of miscarriage.

Women with hyperthyroidism or hypothyroidism have greater risks for miscarriage. Obese and underweight women are more likely to suffer from miscarriages. Women who've smoked and active smokers miscarry more and women who drink excessive amounts of alcohol tend to miscarry more. Patients with viral hepatitis and patients with syphilis have a higher rate of miscarriage. Those who have large uterine fibroids, which tend to get bigger with age, can increase the risk of a first trimester miscarriage. Women suffering from autoimmune diseases, chronic kidney diseases, diabetes, and polycystic ovarian syndrome seem to miscarry more.

Other things that can increase the miscarriage rate include taking certain over-the-counter painkillers, having an exposure to heavy metals, ionizing radiation, and organic solvents, and working in certain manufacturing companies. Environmental toxins of all types can increase the chances of having a miscarriage. Even something as simple as back-to-back pregnancies with less than six months between a current conception and a previous pregnancy can increase the preterm birth rate and the rate of miscarriage. While these risk factors are statistically significant, they don't explain the totality of what causes a miscarriage.

Placenta Previa

In a normal pregnancy, the placenta is located on the upper portion of the uterus. In cases of placenta previa, the placenta has attached to the lower part of the uterus and is completely or partly occluding the opening of the cervix. This is an obstetric complication that happens in about one out of every two hundred vaginal deliveries and seems to happen at a higher risk in women who've had scarring of the uterus from past pregnancies. Fibroid tumors of the uterus and prior surgeries to the uterus increase the chances of having a placenta previa.

Figure 10 indicates what placenta previa looks like:

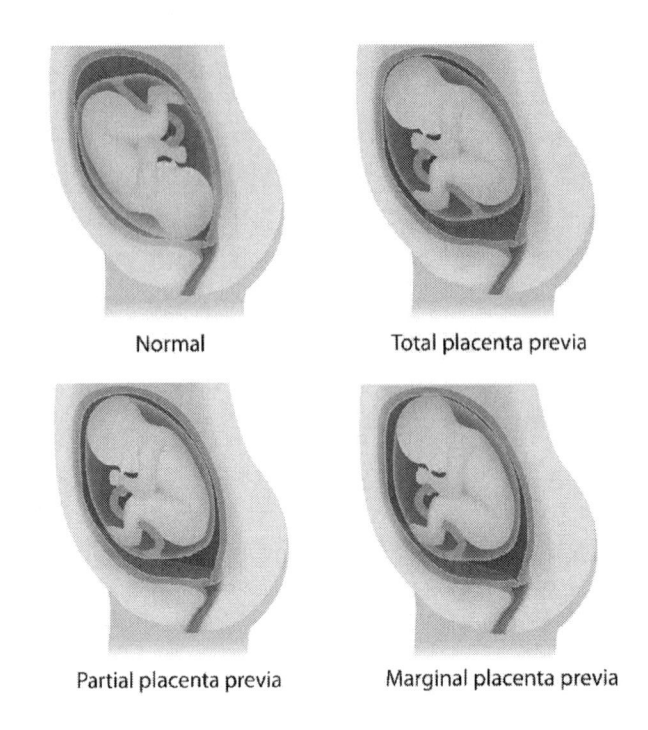

Figure 10

The major symptoms associated with placenta previa include bright red vaginal bleeding unassociated with any type of pelvic or abdominal pain. The bleeding can come on spontaneously or can come on after sexual intercourse. An ultrasound can confirm the presence of a low-lying placenta. Sometimes the placenta rises out of the way of the cervix as the pregnancy progresses but, if it doesn't rise high enough or if it covers the internal os, a cesarean section is necessary as a vaginal delivery is impossible. The act of uterine contractions and cervical dilatation during a vaginal delivery would cause premature separation of the placenta and fetal hypoxia or fetal demise.

A complete placenta previa is defined as having a placenta that completely covers the internal os of the cervix. If the placenta doesn't completely cover the cervical os but is within two centimeters of it, this is called a marginal placenta previa. Both a complete placenta previa and a marginal placenta previa carry a significant risk of hemorrhaging, particularly if the cervix begins to open in the late third trimester. Mortality has been known to occur in both the mother and the fetus in cases where hemorrhaging couldn't be controlled.

Some women aren't discovered to have a placenta previa until the onset of labor. About a third of women will bleed before thirty weeks' gestation, while forty-four percent will bleed after thirty weeks' gestation. When women have documented evidence of placenta previa, almost eighty percent of these women will be symptomatic with bleeding at some point in their pregnancy, usually in the late second or third trimester. Preterm deliveries are a common complication of placenta previa, with nearly half of all pregnancies ending prior to thirty-seven weeks' gestation.

The treatment of placenta previa is most successful when the attending physician anticipates and is prepared to handle a massive hemorrhage. Things like sewing over the placental implantation site, ligating the uterine arteries, ligating the internal iliac arteries, packing the vagina with gauze, and a cesarean hysterectomy are a few of the drastic measures that must be performed to control the hemorrhage and salvage the life of the mother and possibly the fetus.

In cases of a marginal placenta previa that is handled with a vaginal delivery, the delivery can be complicated by severe hemorrhaging at the site of the placental implantation so, even if the delivery is successful, postpartum hemorrhaging can be the unintended outcome. The medical treatments that help this problem include giving methylergonovine maleate or Methergine, prostaglandin F2 alpha, concentrated oxytocin, or misoprostol. These things will help stimulate uterine contractions, overcoming uterine atony, and will possibly correct the problem of hemorrhaging at the site of the placental attachment. Regardless of the treatment given to correct the bleeding, there is often massive blood loss and the need for large amounts of blood products.

Preeclampsia and Eclampsia

The common term for preeclampsia is toxemia or pregnancy-induced hypertension. The main features are high blood pressure, proteinuria, and fluid retention, usually occurring in the third trimester. Unchecked preeclampsia can lead to maternal seizures, in which case the condition is called eclampsia. This can be an obstetrical emergency with the possibility of maternal coma and maternal death.

No one knows the exact cause of preeclampsia. It seems to be more common among women who are in their first pregnancy. About seven to ten percent of pregnancies are complicated by preeclampsia. Most women with the disorder are symptomatic with severe edema of the face and hands, headache, dizziness, high blood pressure, decreased urine output, abdominal pain, blurry vision, and irritability.

As mentioned, it usually happens in the third trimester but can happen as early as twenty weeks' gestation or as late as six weeks' postpartum. While the full range of symptoms have just been described, some women only have hypertension and proteinuria that is only found on physical examination. The classical definition of preeclampsia is having a systolic blood pressure higher than one hundred forty millimeters Hg or a diastolic blood pressure greater than ninety millimeters Hg on at least two occasions and at least four hours apart. A single reading of 160/110 also qualifies as being consistent with preeclampsia. The diagnosis is only confirmed by doing a urine dipstick showing at least 1+ proteinuria or a total of 0.3 grams of protein collected in the urine over a twenty-four-hour period.

Severe preeclampsia is defined as having a blood pressure reading of 160/110 on at least two occasions, the finding of elevated liver enzymes, severe right upper quadrant abdominal pain, worsening renal function with a documented rise in serum creatinine, neurological symptoms, visual disturbances, pulmonary edema, and thrombocytopenia (with a platelet count of less than one hundred thousand cells per microliter). In some cases, preeclampsia can have all the previously-mentioned symptoms in the absence of proteinuria.

The two main complications of preeclampsia are eclampsia, which means there is the new finding of tonic-clonic seizures, and HELLP syndrome, which stands for hemolysis, elevated liver enzymes, and low platelets. Either of these complications can be associated with severe maternal morbidity and mortality.

There are many risk factors for preeclampsia. The main risk factors are having no prior pregnancies, being older than forty years of age, being African-American, having chronic hypertension, having chronic renal disease, having antiphospholipid syndrome, and having a family history of the disorder. Being diabetic and being obese are minor risk factors for preeclampsia. Pregnancies complicated by multiple gestation have a greater risk for preeclampsia in the mother. Rare genetic problems, such as being homozygous for the angiotensinogen gene or being heterozygous for the angiotensinogen gene will raise the suspicion for developing preeclampsia.

All women suspected of having preeclampsia should have a CBC, serum alanine aminotransferase level, serum aspartate aminotransferase level, serum creatinine, uric acid, and twenty-four-hour urine collection for protein and creatinine evaluation. If HELLP syndrome is suspected, a peripheral blood smear will show thrombocytopenia and there will be abnormalities of the serum lactate dehydrogenase level and the serum indirect bilirubin level. Coagulation studies are also performed but are usually of less importance because, if bleeding is likely to be present, it is usually due to a low platelet count and not to clotting factor deficiencies.

A CT scan of the head is done if there is clinical suspicion of an intracerebral hemorrhage from uncontrolled hypertension. CT scans of the head should also be done if the headache is focal in nature, if there are focal neurological deficits, if there are prolonged seizures, or if the diagnosis of eclampsia is not clear. Other imaging studies performed include a sonogram to assess the health of the fetus. Cardiotocography, which is the typical fetal non-stress test can be done to assure ongoing fetal health and wellbeing.

The only real cure for preeclampsia is delivery of the fetus. If there is preeclampsia and a lack of severe features, the obstetrician can wait until after thirty-seven weeks' gestation. If the disease is severe and the fetus isn't yet mature, the woman is hospitalized, placed on bedrest, and monitored for complications with corticosteroids given to enhance fetal lung maturity. Severe preeclampsia that threatens the life of the mother or the fetus generally warrants the induction of labor after thirty-four weeks' gestation. The severity of the disease needs to be directly weighed against the risks of having a preterm infant. The priority in such cases is to control the blood pressure, prevent seizures, and deliver an infant that will be viable upon its birth.

While caring for a woman with preeclampsia, the indications for an urgent delivery include having a non-reassuring fetal stress test, ruptured membranes, uncontrolled hypertension, oligohydramnios, severe intrauterine growth restriction, oliguria, elevated serum creatinine, pulmonary edema, maternal hypoxia, severe headache, HELLP syndrome, eclampsia, severe thrombocytopenia, placental abruption, and unexplained bleeding.

One of the main goals of treating preeclampsia is the prevention of seizures. The basic airway, breathing, and circulation procedures need to be followed and IV magnesium sulfate must be given for the prevention of seizures and the management of active seizures. Magnesium sulfate should be given as a bolus with an intravenous drip of the substance for at least twenty-four hours after the last seizure. All patients with preeclampsia need prophylaxis with magnesium sulfate. Second line agents for refractory seizures include phenytoin and lorazepam.

The second goal for the management of preeclampsia is the treatment of the hypertension itself. The goal is to keep the blood pressure at or below 140/90 using things like hydralazine, labetalol, nifedipine, or sodium nitroprusside, which should be reserved for refractory situations. Even though there is peripheral edema, diuretics should not be given, and aggressive volume resuscitation should be avoided as this can cause secondary pulmonary edema. Most women will need central venous pressure monitoring to maintain homeostasis in the cardiovascular system.

Most patients with preeclampsia will suffer from a transient episode of oliguria after delivery and should have ongoing management with magnesium sulfate until twenty-four hours after childbirth. Liver function testing and platelet counts should be followed and should be normal before discharge. Ongoing hypertension can be managed with oral labetalol or oral nifedipine. The blood pressure should be expected to normalize by the twelfth postpartum week unless the woman is suffering from undiagnosed essential hypertension.

Key Takeaways

- Obstetrical complications can include problems with the placenta, with things like placenta previa and placental abruption.
- There can be pregnancy complications manifesting as polyhydramnios or too much amniotic fluid and oligohydramnios or too little amniotic fluid.
- Miscarriages and fetal demise are obstetrical complications that result in the death of the fetus only, while an ectopic pregnancy can result in the death of the fetus and the mother.
- Preeclampsia and eclampsia are obstetrical conditions that have life-threatening complications for both the mother and the fetus.

Quiz

1. The woman you manage has a pregnancy complicated by polyhydramnios. What is considered a risk factor for this complication?
   a. Fetal obstructive uropathy
   b. Fetal gastrointestinal atresia
   c. Maternal uncontrolled diabetes mellitus
   d. Single umbilical artery

Answer: c. in cases of uncontrolled maternal diabetes mellitus, there can be the secondary finding of polyhydramnios. The other choices are risk factors for oligohydramnios.

2. What is the major fetal complication seen in pregnancies complicated by oligohydramnios?
   a. Duodenal atresia
   b. Fetal kidney failure
   c. Fetal obstructive uropathy
   d. Lack of fetal pulmonary development

Answer: d. With a lack of amniotic fluid, the fetal lungs are unable to practice breathing in utero and there will be the complication of a lack of fetal pulmonary development. The other choices are causes of, not complications of oligohydramnios.

3. What is the most significant potential outcome of untreated placental abruption?
   a. Preterm labor
   b. Premature rupture of the membranes

c. Maternal anemia
d. Fetal hypoxia

Answer: d. As the placental abruption increases, there will be a lack of contact between the placenta and the maternal circulation which results in fetal hypoxia and eventual fetal death.

4. What is the most important management strategy in treating a woman with symptomatic placenta previa?
    a. Giving intravenous corticosteroids to enhance fetal lung maturity
    b. Preparing for a massive maternal hemorrhage
    c. Giving platelets and fresh frozen plasma to correct a coagulopathy
    d. Giving intravenous antibiotics to prevent chorioamnionitis

Answer: b. The biggest complication of placenta previa is massive maternal hemorrhage so any management of this condition needs to have the strategy of preparing for this possibility.

5. Which is the most common cause of intrauterine fetal loss after twenty weeks' gestation?
    a. Maternal toxin exposure
    b. Incompetent cervix
    c. Fetal chromosomal abnormality
    d. Fetal cardiac anomaly

Answer: b. The most common cause of intrauterine fetal loss after twenty weeks' gestation is an incompetent cervix.

6. What is the best treatment strategy for an ectopic pregnancy that has not yet ruptured the fallopian tube?
    a. Laparoscopic removal of the products of conception
    b. Laparotomy and excision of the fallopian tube
    c. Observance of the HCG levels for a natural decline as the pregnancy resolves itself
    d. Methotrexate to dissolve the products of conception and maintain tubal patency

Answer: d. Methotrexate is an effective treatment choice for an unruptured fallopian tube ectopic pregnancy. It may help resorb the products of conception before the fallopian tube ruptures, which also maintains tube patency.

7. What is considered a severe manifestation of preeclampsia?
    a. Blurry vision
    b. Headache
    c. HELLP syndrome
    d. Peripheral edema

Answer: c. HELLP syndrome involves severe injury to the liver and thrombocytopenia, which is a severe complication of preeclampsia. The other symptoms are a part of preeclampsia but may be present with mild and severe preeclampsia.

8. You are managing a pregnancy complicated by preeclampsia. What is the major goal of the treatment of the disorder?
    a. Prevention of eclampsia

b. Providing corticosteroids to enhance fetal lung maturity
   c. Preventing renal insufficiency in the mother
   d. Preventing oligohydramnios

Answer: a. A major goal in the treatment of preeclampsia is the prevention of eclampsia, which can have life-threatening complications for the mother and fetus.

9. Which can be considered a major risk factor for a first trimester miscarriage?
   a. Maternal age greater than forty
   b. Primiparous mother
   c. Vitamin A deficiency
   d. Twin pregnancy

Answer: a. A maternal age greater than forty is a major risk factor for a first trimester miscarriage with almost a third of these ending in a miscarriage.

10. You are managing the care of a woman with preeclampsia. What is the best treatment you can offer to prevent the onset of eclampsia?
    a. Intravenous nitroprusside
    b. Intravenous magnesium sulfate
    c. Intravenous labetalol
    d. Oral nifedipine

Answer: b. While there are many good treatments for a patient's hypertension when treating preeclampsia, the only way to prevent eclampsia is to give intravenous magnesium sulfate until the danger of seizures is past.

Chapter 9: Infections in Pregnancy

While pregnant women can get any type of infection, the main infections that are clinically important in treating a pregnant woman include the various sexually transmitted diseases, uterine infections, cervical infections, and vaginal infections—each of which has the capacity to affect the fetus.

Group B Streptococcus

Group B Streptococcus is the most common cause of life-threatening infections in the neonate and can also have an adverse effect on the pregnant woman. It should be noted that Group B streptococcus can be found as a normal part of the mouth, rectal, and vaginal flora and only cause infection under certain circumstances. This means that the mother may be colonized but may not know it until the infection inadvertently affects the newborn in what can be a very serious infection.

Women in pregnancy can get bacterial cystitis, chorioamnionitis, endometritis, and stillbirth if she is infected with Group B streptococcus. Bacteremia from the bacterium can lead to meningitis or endocarditis. Postpartum women have the potential to get urinary tract infections or even abscesses in the pelvis if the infection becomes extremely entrenched in her pelvic structures.

Newborns become colonized with Group B streptococcus at the time they pass through the birth canal and can have an early-onset Group B Streptococcal infection prior to the age of seven days, with a mean age at presentation being about twelve hours. The main clinical syndromes seen are non-focal sepsis, bacterial pneumonia, or neonatal meningitis. Late onset disease in infants can occur as late as ninety days after birth, with an average age of about one month. Babies who survive the initial infection can suffer complications, such as hearing loss, vision loss, learning disabilities, or other neurological complications.

According to the Centers for Disease Control and Prevention, all pregnant women should be screened at thirty-five to thirty-seven weeks' gestation for Group B streptococcus with a rectal and vaginal swab. The best place to perform a culture is at the vaginal introitus, just inside the hymen, and in the rectum, just beyond the anal sphincter. Cultures of the cervix, perianal skin, perirectal tissues, or perineum should not be obtained. A speculum should not be used at any time during the culture process.

If the Group B streptococcus culture is positive, the woman will need treatment for the infection during labor. If there are no cultures available, high risk women should receive antibiotic prophylaxis anyway. High risk women include those with a previous Group B streptococcal infection, bacteriuria during pregnancy that cultured positive for Group B strep, preterm delivery, duration of ruptured membranes longer than eighteen hours, and a fever during labor of more than 100.4 degrees Fahrenheit. Any woman who screened negative within five weeks of going into labor do not require treatment.

Treatment of Group B streptococcus during labor include intravenous penicillin or ampicillin in women who are not allergic to penicillin. If allergic to penicillin, the culture should be sent for sensitivities, although most streptococcal infections are sensitive to intravenous cefazolin. Women with anaphylaxis from penicillin should receive IV clindamycin or erythromycin. IV vancomycin is another possibility if the allergy status of the woman is not known. Even with preventative antibiotics, the newborn should be monitored carefully for infection.

Urinary Tract Infections

Asymptomatic bacterial colonization of the urinary tract can develop in as many as fifteen percent of women who are pregnant and can lead to complications such as pyelonephritis, premature labor, and urosepsis. This means that all pregnant woman should have a screening test including a urine culture at least once during the time of pregnancy and should be treated, even if there are no symptoms. Significant bacteriuria is defined as having more than a hundred thousand colony-forming units of any single organism in a clean-catch specimen.

The treatment of urinary tract infections in pregnancy may be empiric, followed by selecting an antibiotic that will be effective against the organism as identified by sensitivity testing. The main antibiotics that can be used in pregnancy are sulfonamide drugs, augmentin, amoxicillin, cephalexin, and nitrofurantoin. It should be noted that sulfonamides in the last few weeks of gestation may lead to severe jaundice in the newborn, so this should be avoided. Trimethoprim cannot be used in the first trimester as it has been found to be teratogenic to a slight degree. Patients or fetuses who have Glucose-6-phosphodiesterase deficiency cannot take nitrofurantoin.

A course of seven days of antibiotics should be given, which will treat both symptomatic and asymptomatic disease. One day treatments are not recommended. Recurrences of bladder infections in pregnancy will require treatment with a single dose of cephalexin or nitrofurantoin, especially of infections are common after sexual intercourse.

Other than the need to avoid certain antibiotics, the treatment of pyelonephritis in pregnant women is no different that treating a woman who is pregnant. If the situation is mild, outpatient management can be done. If the patient has severe symptoms or possible sepsis, inpatient treatment and IV hydration are necessary to avoid dehydration. Follow up urine cultures should continue for the rest of the pregnancy with prophylactic antibiotics given for recurrent bacteriuria.

Bacterial Vaginosis

Research has shown that bacterial vaginosis during pregnancy does have some complications. It is associated with an increased chance of having a preterm birth and of having an infant that is small for gestational age. Premature rupture of the membranes before thirty-seven weeks' gestation and postpartum uterine infections are also possible after childbirth. There is some indication of an increased risk of second trimester miscarriages in women with bacterial vaginosis. Even so, the clear majority of women with bacterial vaginosis will have completely normal pregnancies and up to half of these infections will go away spontaneously.

One significant risk of having bacterial vaginosis is that the woman is more susceptible to getting various types of sexually transmitted infections, including HIV, gonorrhea, chlamydia, and other STDs. In women who aren't pregnant, bacterial vaginosis has been connected to a higher than normal risk of getting pelvic inflammatory disease and post-operative infections following gynecological surgery. Pelvic inflammatory disease can happen in pregnancy, but it is a relatively rare occurrence.

During pregnancy, women with bacterial vaginosis will have no symptoms at least half the time. The only major symptoms noted are a whitish or grayish discharge that smells like fish or has other unpleasant odors. It is most obviously smelled shortly after intercourse. Dysuria or genital irritation can occur but is not as common of a problem with this infection.

Women without symptoms and who have low-risk pregnancies are not screened for bacterial vaginosis. Research indicates that treating asymptomatic pregnant women for bacterial vaginosis doesn't alter the chances of a preterm birth unless the woman has already had a preterm birth in the past.

Women at high risk for having a preterm birth may be screened for bacterial vaginosis at the first prenatal visit, even if they have no symptoms. Treating these infections early in pregnancy may or may not reduce the risk of preterm birth as the infection can come back at any time during pregnancy. Because of this, experts are conflicted about whether the infection should be screened for, even in high risk women.

The treatment of bacterial vaginosis is antibiotics that can be taken orally and are safe during pregnancy. The treatment of choice is metronidazole or clindamycin. There is no need to treat the sexual partner of the pregnant woman. The entire course of antibiotics needs to be taken, even after the symptoms have resolved.

The biggest problem is that thirty percent of women will have symptoms of bacterial vaginosis again within three months after treatment. This is because getting rid of the infectious agents does not replace the good bacteria in the vagina so there is an increased chance of redeveloping the infection.

Listeriosis

Listeriosis is not a common infection in pregnant women, which is complicated by its common underdiagnoses. It can cause neonatal sepsis, and accounts for about two thousand five hundred infections in neonates each year in the US. About five hundred babies die from the disease every year. Fortunately, the rate of this infection is decreasing because of increased public awareness regarding what a woman should do to avoid getting colonization during pregnancy. About twenty percent of active maternal infections will lead to a fetal loss.

Listeria monocytogenes is a Gram-positive bacterium with both aerobic and anaerobic abilities. The organism can be found in dirt and water and can be carried by animals. The meat from these animals is processed into lunch meat and other processed meats. Unpasteurized milk and raw foods can also be sources of listeriosis.

Pregnant women have twenty times increased risk of developing bacteremia with the listeria organism. About a third of all cases of listeriosis reported to the CDC involve pregnant women, most of which have the infection in the third trimester. This is unfortunately when the woman's cell-mediated immune system is the most impaired. The infection is caused by eating food that is contaminated by the bacterium although direct contact with animals can also cause the infection.

The organism, can be found in dirt and water. Vegetables can become contaminated with the bacterium if the grower used fertilizer made from manure. The other main source, that of processed meats from contaminated animals. Rarer causes of listeriosis include contaminated cheeses, which can cause sporadic outbreaks of the infection.

The most common findings on clinical presentation of listeriosis in women who are pregnant is symptomatic bacteremia. Central nervous system infections are common among non-pregnant individuals with the disease but do not seem to play a big role in pregnancy-related disease. To make matters more complicated, pregnant women with the disease often have no symptoms or only a febrile illness that they mistake for influenza. Even in asymptomatic women, the risk for preterm birth is elevated as is the risk to the neonate. Stillbirths from listeriosis have also been documented.

Placental transfer of the listeria bacterium to the fetus can result in chorioamnionitis and a secondary septic miscarriage. Babies closer to term will not miscarry but can die in utero or be born prematurely. The fetus and newborn can have septicemia, meningoencephalitis, or disseminated disease with micro-abscesses and granulomatous disease. As mentioned, about twenty percent of infections around the time of childbirth will result in death to the newborn or stillbirth. The chances of becoming infected as a newborn with a listeriosis-positive mother is about two-thirds. The mortality rate in these babies is as high as fifty percent. Babies can be affected shortly after birth or can develop a meningitis from listeriosis at about two to four weeks of age.

Routine screening for this bacterium is not recommended in pregnant women as colonization with the bacterium in the gastrointestinal tract or vaginal canal does not increase the risk of developing a symptomatic infection during pregnancy. Symptomatic women in pregnancy can be diagnosed by doing a blood culture, which will grow out listeria, particularly in feverish women. If the woman has had listeria in pregnancy, cultures should be obtained from the meconium of the infant, the infant's eyes, the infant's nose, the infant's urine, the infant's blood, the cerebrospinal fluid, the placenta, or the mother's lochia.

According to the US Centers for Disease Control and Prevention, the best way to avoid listeriosis in neonates is to prevent the woman from becoming colonized by the bacterium. All raw food from animal sources should be pasteurized and all raw vegetables should be washed prior to ingestion. Uncooked meats and vegetables should be separated from cooked foods. Unpasteurized foods from milk products should not be eaten. After cooking, all utensils, hands, and cutting boards should be thoroughly scrubbed with a bactericidal agent. Foods that are perishable should be eaten as soon as they are washed.

A listeriosis infection can be diagnosed by doing a culture that grows out Listeria monocytogenes in the blood or cerebrospinal fluid of the mother or neonate. There is no serological testing for this illness and cultures of the stool are impractical as they aren't very specific or sensitive for the disease.

The main treatment for listeriosis is intravenous ampicillin, given at two grams intravenously every four hours. Penicillin can be given intravenously every four hours as well. If patients are allergic to these, trimethoprim/sulfamethoxazole is a suitable alternative but is not usually recommended in the third trimester of pregnancy.

Syphilis

It is crucial that syphilis be diagnosed and treated as early as possible in pregnancy to prevent untoward complications associated with syphilis infections in pregnancy. Untreated primary or secondary syphilis among pregnant women may lead to congenital syphilis in the neonate about half the time. This is not a very common infection in pregnancy, with only about four hundred fifty cases of the disorder identified in the US per year. The main thing that leads to congenital syphilis is no routine prenatal care.

The organism that causes syphilis is a spirochete known as Treponema pallidum. There are several stages to the disease and the type of complication that happens depends on the stage of the maternal disease the neonate is exposed to. The earlier during the disease, the higher is the risk of morbidity in the infant. Untreated primary or secondary syphilitic disease in pregnancy leads to a fetal infection nearly always. Infection of the fetus prior to the fourth month of gestation is not very common. Later exposures can result in a late spontaneous abortion, stillbirth, neonatal infection, neonatal death, or an infection in the infant that is older than a newborn.

The clinical course of syphilis in pregnancy is about the same as it is in non-pregnancy cases. The initial finding is that of a hard, painless red ulcer that generally forms on the vulva, cervix, or female vagina. After this, the woman can have secondary syphilis, which involves a rash on the palms of the hands and the soles of the feet. Fever, swollen lymph nodes, and joint pain can be part of this stage of syphilis. The latent stage of syphilis often is asymptomatic and, while it cannot be passed to a sexual partner, the woman can pass the disease on to their fetus during childbirth or in utero. A third of women will develop tertiary syphilis, which can damage the heart. At any stage, there can be CNS or eye complications, including neurosyphilis.

Even though syphilis is uncommon, all women are screened for syphilis with a rapid plasmin reagin test, which is a serological test for syphilis. The earlier in pregnancy a syphilis infection is determined to be present, the better the treatment will be. Therefore, the screening test is done at the first prenatal visit. In high risk patients, a repeat serology study is done at twenty-eight weeks' gestation.

As mentioned, screening is done by a blood test. The main nontreponemal antibody testing done for screening purposes are the rapid plasmin reagin test and the Venereal Disease Research Laboratory test or VRDL. These are very sensitive tests but aren't specific to syphilis, with an increased risk of falsely positive tests. Any positive screening test should be followed up with a specific anti-treponemal antibody test, such as the T pallidum (MHA-TP) test or the fluorescent treponemal antibody absorption test or FTA-ABS test. These do not indicate an active infection as they are always going to be positive in cases where the woman had an active infection in the past. The best way to document an active infection is to take a sample from a visible lesion in primary syphilis and do a dark-field examination under the microscope, which will identify the treponemal organism. Because most women in pregnancy have no identifiable lesions, the only way they can be tested is through serological testing.

Once syphilis is diagnosed, the woman should be tested for other sexually transmitted diseases, including HIV disease, while she is being started on anti-syphilis treatment. The treatment for the disorder in pregnancy is a single dose of more than two million units of intramuscular penicillin, which is effective in primary, secondary, and early latent disease. A second dose should be given a week after the first dose in women who are in the third trimester or who have secondary syphilis. Late latent syphilis needs more aggressive management with three doses of benzathine penicillin given intramuscularly three weeks apart from one another. If a follow up quantitative VDRL test shows a four-fold increase in the titer, the patient should be treated all over again and should have a lumbar puncture to make sure she doesn't have neurosyphilis.

Unfortunately, penicillin is the only drug available for use in pregnant women with syphilis. Penicillin reaches the highest concentration in amniotic fluid when compared to other drugs, which may not reach this crucial part of the fetus and surrounding fluid. Penicillin-allergic women require desensitization so they can receive appropriate treatment. Unfortunately, other choices, such as erythromycin and tetracycline cannot be used as erythromycin won't prevent congenital syphilis and tetracycline can't be given in pregnancy. Ceftriaxone and azithromycin haven't been adequately researched and not recommended testaments.

The biggest risk in giving penicillin to pregnant women with an early case of syphilis is the development of an unusual reaction, known as a Jarish-Herzheimer reaction. It involves the onset of premature uterine contractions, a possible preterm birth, and a premature infant. Even so, the treatment is necessary, and the complication should be managed like any other preterm labor complication.

Chlamydia

Chlamydia trachomatous is an unusual pathogen that is the most common bacterial sexually transmitted disease in the United States and continues to be a major cause of pregnancy complications and neonatal complications. About seventy-five percent of women with this infection have no symptoms, even when the infection is seriously affecting their reproductive tract. Symptomatic women can get cervicitis, endometritis, acute urethral syndrome, and acute pelvic inflammatory disease. Pregnant women can also get chorioamnionitis, gestational hemorrhaging, and postpartum endometritis if not identified and treated.

The usual way an infant contract the disease is through the birth canal in the second stage of labor. Neonatal chlamydia infections generally affect the eyes, causing a conjunctivitis known as ophthalmia neonatorum. Pneumonia from chlamydia can also affect newborns. For this reason, all pregnant mothers need chlamydia screening as early in pregnancy as possible. High-risk mothers and mothers under the age of twenty-five should have a repeat culture done of the cervix at some point in the third trimester. Women who have infections in the first trimester should be rechecked three to six months later, even if they have been treated for the condition.

The best screening methods for chlamydia include the nucleic acid amplification test or NAAT. This is done on a urine specimen or on a specimen taken by a swab placed on the cervix. An endocervical swab can be cultured for chlamydia and direct fluorescent antibody testing, enzyme immunoassay testing, or unamplified nucleic acid testing can be done if an endocervical swab cannot be obtained.

The main treatment strategies for chlamydia include giving azithromycin, which is the first line agent. Other antibiotics that can be given second line include amoxicillin and erythromycin. While tetracycline and fluoroquinolones will kill chlamydia infections, they cannot be given to pregnant women. A three-week follow up test should be done to make sure the infection has cleared.

Gonorrhea

Gonorrhea infections can be tricky in that they cause no symptoms in up to half of all patients, so it needs to be screened for in early pregnancy. Gonorrhea screening is often done at the first prenatal visit along with chlamydia testing as these infections often go together. Gonorrhea is the second most common sexually transmitted disease in pregnancy. Pregnant women can technically pass the infection to the infant in utero but usually pass it on to the baby as the baby passes through the birth canal. The resulting infection can be life-threatening. Therefore, early detection is warranted in pregnancy.

The cause of gonorrhea is Neisseria gonorrhoeae, which is a gram-negative diplococcal bacterium. It is an STD passed from one sexual partner to another and is transmitted vertically through the cervix and vagina. There is no evidence that it can pass through the placenta from the woman's bloodstream. Gonorrhea in women can infect the uterus, fallopian tubes, cervix, and ovaries. Ectopic pregnancies and infertility can be secondary complications of untreated infections.

Most pregnant women with gonorrhea have no symptoms but some will have endocervicitis, premature rupture of the amniotic sac, chorioamnionitis, septic abortion, preterm birth, postpartum sepsis, and intrauterine growth restriction in the neonate. The frequency of pelvic inflammatory disease in pregnancy is less than in non-pregnant women because the uterus is relatively immune to the passage of the bacterium through the cervix during pregnancy. Proctitis is another complication of pregnancies affected by gonorrhea and can be found in up to half of all women in pregnancy who have the disorder. In some cases, the organism can only be identified by means of a rectal swab and must be a part of the screening process.

Neonates exposed to gonorrhea at the time of birth may have the development of an acute conjunctivitis known as ophthalmia neonatorum, sepsis, arthritis, and/or meningitis. The most important preventive measure for the development of neonatal gonococcal disease is the screening and subsequent antibiotic use in pregnant women before giving birth. Disseminated gonococcal disease is a possibility in pregnancy, with symptoms including a characteristic rash and polyarthralgias that migrate from join to joint. The rash can be seen over the distal joints and is both vesicular and pustular in nature. These women are sick and often have a fever.

Because pregnant women with gonorrhea are often asymptomatic, it is vital that they be screened early in the pregnancy. The recommendation is to screen women who are at high risk for STDs by doing an endocervical swab and culturing the swab for the gonorrhea bacterium. The CDC goes as far as recommending that all women be screened for the infection in the third trimester, regardless of risk. There is a NAAT test and a nucleic acid hybridization test available for gonorrhea infection surveillance, but the culture is the gold standard.

The treatment of gonorrhea can be complex because it has the potential to develop antibiotic resistances quite easily. Quinolone-resistant strains are found to a great degree in the United States and in other parts of the world, and not recommended as a first line agent. They are also contraindicated in pregnancy. Cephalosporins are the first line treatment for gonorrhea. For gonorrheal cervicitis, for example, two hundred fifty milligrams of ceftriaxone are given intramuscularly as a single injection along with oral azithromycin at a dose of one gram all at one time. Women allergic to cephalosporins can receive azithromycin at two grams given orally. All patients with gonorrhea need treatment for chlamydia as well even if no chlamydia testing was done or if the organism didn't grow in a culture medium. The existence of coinfections is high so double treatment for both organisms is recommended.

Key Takeaways

- Infections in pregnancy have the potential to be passed to the fetus in utero either by ascending spreads of the infection through the cervix or by being passed through the placenta from the maternal circulation.
- Bacterial vaginosis may have no symptoms but can cause mild pregnancy complications affecting the fetus, so it should be treated when found in pregnancy.
- Syphilis can cause severe neurological complications in neonates, so it needs to be screened for in early pregnancy.
- Infections with gonorrhea and chlamydia often go together so they are treated together if either one of the infections is identified.
- Listeriosis is an infection from processed meats and unwashed produce that is only significant if it is an infection that occurs in pregnancy.

Quiz

1. The woman is in her first trimester and believes she has bacterial vaginosis. What is the most common symptom of the infection that would alert the woman she has the infection?
    a. Dysuria
    b. Perineal burning
    c. Low pelvic pain
    d. Malodorous vaginal discharge

Answer: d. There are very few symptoms associated with bacterial vaginosis. The main symptom noted by women is a malodorous vaginal discharge that often smells like fish.

2. You are discussing neonatal infections with a mother who is about to give birth. In discussing this, you tell her the most common serious infection in her newborn will likely be what?
    a. Listeriosis
    b. Group B streptococcus sepsis
    c. Gonorrhea sepsis
    d. Neurosyphilis

Answer: b. The most common serious infection in neonates is group B streptococcus sepsis. The other infections are much less likely to occur in neonates.

3. You are advising a woman in her first trimester of how to avoid contraction Listeriosis. What is the main thing you say to adviser about avoiding the infection?
    a. Stay away from cow's milk
    b. Eat only cooked vegetables
    c. Stay away from processed lunch meats
    d. Avoid eating at restaurants

Answer: c. As the Listeria infection can come from processed lunch meats that haven't been properly handled, pregnant women should avoid eating processed lunch meats.

4. You are evaluating a woman for the possibility of having syphilis while pregnant. What screening test is most used for this purpose?
    a. Rapid plasma reagin test
    b. Anti-treponemal antibody test
    c. T pallidum test
    d. Chancre culture for treponemal organisms

Answer: a. The main screening test for syphilis is the rapid plasma reagin test. The other tests can be confirmatory or aren't used in the screening of patients for syphilis.

5. A woman is found to have a positive culture for chlamydia in the middle of the third trimester. What is a first line agent for the treatment of this condition in pregnancy?
    a. Azithromycin
    b. Amoxicillin
    c. Erythromycin
    d. Ciprofloxacin

Answer: a. Azithromycin is the first line agent for the treatment of chlamydia in pregnancy. The other choices are not first line agents or are contraindicated in pregnancy.

6. Why is a pregnant woman with a positive gonorrhea culture given both a cephalosporin and azithromycin?
    a. Because there are a lot of drug resistances in gonorrheal infections.
    b. Because the two antibiotics work synergistically together.
    c. Because this enhances compliance with treatment.
    d. Because there is a high likelihood of a concomitant chlamydia infection that needs to be treated as well with azithromycin.

Answer: d. Women with a positive gonorrhea culture in pregnancy have a high risk of a concomitant chlamydia infection so empiric coverage for chlamydia is done even if it was not cultured or otherwise identified.

7. What is the most serious complication of a neonatal infection with gonorrhea?
    a. Ophthalmia neonatorum
    b. Gonorrheal myocarditis
    c. Gonorrheal meningitis
    d. Gonorrheal conjunctivitis

Answer: c. The most serious complication of a neonatal infection with gonorrhea is gonorrheal meningitis, which can develop shortly after birth.

8. Pregnant women seem to have a higher risk of urinary tract infections and pyelonephritis. What percentage of pregnant women will have asymptomatic bacteriuria at some point in their pregnancy?
    a. Five percent

b. Ten percent
  c. Fifteen percent
  d. Twenty-five percent

Answer: c. Up to fifteen percent of pregnant women will have asymptomatic bacteriuria at some point in the pregnancy so cultures of the urine should be performed at least once as part of good prenatal care.

9. What is the most common presentation among pregnant women who have documented Chlamydia?
    a. Dysuria
    b. Cervical bleeding
    c. Yellow vaginal discharge
    d. No symptoms

Answer: d. Up to seventy-five percent of pregnant women with chlamydia will have no symptoms and should evaluated for, even if no symptoms are present.

10. A pregnant mother has given birth and her infant quickly develops meningitis and grows Listeria out of the cerebrospinal fluid. What is the treatment of choice for this neonate?
    a. Intravenous ampicillin
    b. Oral trimethoprim/sulfamethoxazole
    c. Intravenous ciprofloxacin
    d. Intravenous vancomycin

Answer: a. The treatment of choice for a pregnant mother or her infant who have documented listeria infections is to give intravenous ampicillin, particularly for neonatal meningitis.

Chapter 10: Twin Gestation

While most women have only one baby per pregnancy, a fair number of women may carry more than one baby. This can be overwhelming for any couple preparing to have children and there are more risks associated with this type of pregnancy. The common risks and manifestations of a twin pregnancy are discussed in this chapter.

Twin Basic Facts

Twin pregnancies occur to a greater degree among older mothers because they have a unique hormonal environment that causes more than one egg to be released at one time per cycle. If both eggs get fertilized and implant in the uterine cavity, the result is a fraternal twin gestation. Fraternal twins are also found to a greater degree in women undergoing assisted reproductive technology procedures, such as in vitro fertilization. More than one embryo is transferred to the mother's uterus in the hopes that at least one will implant. In some cases, more than one will implant and higher order multiples such as twins, triplets, and quadruplets can be the result.

Figure 11 describes the different types of twin pregnancies:

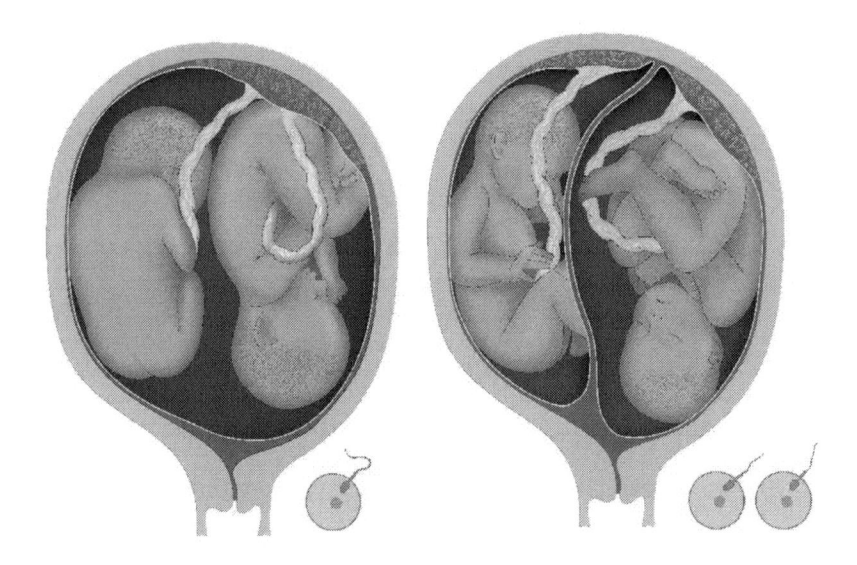

Figure 11

By definition, all fraternal twins come from two separate eggs and two separate sperm. They tend not to look alike any more than two siblings, and it is possible to have a twin of each gender. Each twin has its own placenta and its own amniotic sac. Fraternal twin pregnancies are safer than identical twin pregnancies because there is no sharing of nutrients and blood from a single placenta.

Identical twin pregnancies occur when a single fertilized egg splits in two and two fetuses develop from the split products of gestation. The twins may have the same placenta but usually, each baby has its own amniotic sac. These babies are genetically identical and will be of the same gender. Failure of the fertilized egg or embryo to completely split apart can lead to conjoined twins.

Twin pregnancies are often suspected when the uterus is bigger than normal in the first or second trimester or if there are two separate heartbeats detected. In modern times, a twin pregnancy is always confirmed by an ultrasound that will easily show two fetuses and the characteristics of each fetus. In some cases, a twin pregnancy early in the first trimester is evaluated later and only one baby is found. This is called the vanishing twin syndrome and means that one baby was lost while the other baby survived.

Managing the Twin Gestation

The mother should be seen more frequently for prenatal visits as they are at a higher than normal risk for preterm labor and intrauterine growth restriction of one or both twins. These mothers need more iron, protein, folic acid, and calcium than singleton moms. The mother carrying twins can expect to gain more weight than would be found in a singleton pregnancy. The recommended weight gain for a twin gestation is thirty-seven to fifty-four pounds if the woman was of a normal weight prior to the pregnancy. The caloric intake needs to be about six hundred calories higher than the intake before pregnancy and there will be more restrictions on physical activity and traveling because of the greater risk for preterm labor. Twin pregnancies are often delivered sooner than singleton pregnancies and mothers are generally induced or will have a cesarean section by the thirty-eighth or thirty-ninth week of pregnancy.

Twin Complications

There are complications that should be considered in a twin pregnancy that are not commonly encountered in singleton pregnancies. Mothers with twins have a higher than average chance of having hypertension in pregnancy. Both gestational hypertension and hypertension from preeclampsia occur at a higher rate in twin pregnancies. For this reason, the mother's blood pressure needs to be monitored more carefully if she is carrying twins.

Preterm births are more common in twin pregnancies. The uterus is overly large and is more sensitive to preterm labor and preterm irritability. Steroids are often given when it appears the births are inevitable to maximize lung maturity before delivery. Preterm infants commonly encounter complications after birth, such as visual deficits, premature lungs, digestive problems, intracerebral hemorrhages, and infections. In rare circumstances, one twin is delivered many days before the second twin is delivered in what is known as a delayed interval delivery.

Identical twins can have a problem known as twin-twin transfusion syndrome. This happens when a blood vessel in the placenta connects to the fetuses' circulatory systems. This causes one of the twins to get too much blood, while another twin gets too little blood. This can be a serious complication for both babies that will necessitate a premature delivery to manage this problem.

If the first baby is in the head down position, a vaginal delivery of twins is possible but if the presenting twin is breech, a cesarean section is usually recommended. Cesarean births are almost always recommended in situations where there are higher order multiples than just twins.

The First Trimester in a Twin Pregnancy

The first thirteen weeks are considered the first trimester. The common symptoms seen in a twin pregnancy tend to be more exaggerated because the hormonal milieu is usually higher causing increased nausea, vomiting, and significant first trimester fatigue. The human chorionic gonadotropin level is much higher in a twin gestation and therefore the symptoms of pregnancy are more prominent.

Women carrying twins in the first trimester will look more pregnant than women carrying a singleton pregnancy, as more fetuses cause the uterus to be much larger and rise above the pubic symphysis prior to the twelfth week of gestation. Because the symptoms of a twin pregnancy are more obvious, women with twins tend to see the doctor sooner and are diagnosed as being pregnant with twins sooner than would happen in a singleton pregnancy.

The evaluation of a woman carrying twins in the first trimester shows a rapidly expanding uterus that is large for gestational age. The weight gain is excessive, and the woman has more intense symptoms of nausea and vomiting, extremely tender breasts, more urinary frequency, and extreme fatigue. When the nausea abates, the woman tends to be hungrier than would happen in a singleton pregnancy and the woman will have a greater sensitivity to certain foods and certain smells.

The Second Trimester in a Twin Pregnancy

The second trimester is, by definition, from the fourteenth week to the twenty-seventh week. This is usually better tolerated by women carrying twins, with fewer symptoms than the first trimester. The nausea and fatigue abate to a great degree and the uterus, while large for gestational age, is still of a comfortable size.

During the second trimester, the woman will have renewed energy and will be more optimistic and happy about the pregnancy. The pregnancy is relatively enjoyable, and many women become delighted with the idea of having twins. The shock has worn off and the woman has become accustomed to the idea that she is having twins.

The second trimester is when the woman experiences a greater sense of organization and will begin to plan the pregnancy and her future with her babies. She becomes more emotionally connected to her babies and feels less fearful about the pregnancy. The ultrasound will easily visualize the twins on the monitor and the woman will start feeling the twins moving in the womb. The ultrasound technician may be able to tell if the pregnancy is one of identical twins or fraternal twins and the genders of the babies. The ultrasound that can tell the gender of the twins usually happens between the eighteenth and twentieth week of the pregnancy.

The Third Trimester in a Twin Pregnancy

The third trimester begins at the twenty-eight week of pregnancy and ends at about week forty. This is when it becomes relatively obvious that the woman is carrying twins because she is much larger than a woman with just one baby. Walking around is more difficult and the weight of the uterus may cause a separation of the symphysis pubis, which impacts the woman's ability to walk comfortably. Sleep is less comfortable, and the woman tends to become increasingly sleep deprived.

The fetal movements can be extremely strong and, because the uterine wall is thin, the babies' movements can be seen from an external inspection. Small and petite women carrying twins will have more difficulty breathing as the uterus quickly reaches the xyphoid process. This is the time when the fatigue comes back and the energy levels dip to a new low. Women with twins will have more edema than women with singleton pregnancies and will see the obstetrician on a weekly basis until the time of delivery. Preterm delivery is always a possibility and should be monitored carefully as one of the priority items to follow in a twin gestation in the third trimester.

Risks in a Twin Pregnancy

Twin pregnancies carry a higher risk all around, from the beginning of the first trimester until the day the twins are born. There is a greater chance of pregnancy complications throughout the pregnancy. This means an increased risk of preeclampsia, an increased risk of eclampsia, an increased risk of gestational diabetes, and a higher chance of gestational hypertension. While vaginal deliveries of twins are still possible, the chances of having a primary cesarean section that is planned is higher. There is also the possibility of having one twin delivered vaginally with failure of the second twin to be delivered vaginally, resulting in an urgent cesarean section of the second twin.

Because the risk of preterm birth with twins is higher, twins tend to be born smaller than their singleton counterparts, and each twin will carry all the concomitant complications that go along with being born at a gestational age that is not full term. These babies will have a higher than average chance of spending time in the neonatal intensive care unit or other specialty nursery until they are more fully developed.

Key Takeaways

- Twin pregnancies can involve identical twins or fraternal twins.
- Twin pregnancies involve having more severe first trimester symptoms due to higher HCG levels and higher levels of other pregnancy hormones.
- Twin pregnancies with fraternal twins are safer than twin pregnancies with identical twins because each twin has its own placenta and amniotic sac.
- The most common complication of a twin gestation is prematurity and the complications that go along with being preterm at birth.

Quiz

1. Which is considered a risk factor for having a fraternal twin pregnancy?
    a. Having a history of infertility
    b. Having a history of pelvic inflammatory disease
    c. Being an older mother at the time of pregnancy
    d. Having several previous childbirths

Answer: c. Of the choices given, being an older mother at the time of pregnancy is a risk factor for having fraternal twins as older women are more likely to release more than one egg at a time.

2. Why do women in the first trimester of pregnancy with twins have greater symptoms of nausea and vomiting?
    a. The uterus is bigger and presses on the stomach.
    b. The levels of HCG are higher in twin gestations.
    c. The estradiol level is higher in twin gestations.
    d. The woman is less able to eat healthy foods when she is carrying twins.

Answer: b. HCG levels are directly associated with the level of nausea and vomiting. In pregnancies with twins, the HCG levels are higher than normal pregnancies and the risk of these symptoms is greater.

3. At what point during a twin pregnancy will the pregnant woman feel the most active and have the most energy?
    a. Sixth week gestation
    b. Tenth week gestation
    c. Fifteenth week gestation
    d. Twenty-seventh week gestation

Answer: c. Women in the second trimester of a twin pregnancy tend to feel more energized, with an increase in activity level.

4. When can the ultrasound technician tell the woman in a twin pregnancy what the genders are of her fetuses?
    a. Twelve to fourteen weeks
    b. Fourteen to sixteen weeks
    c. Sixteen to eighteen weeks
    d. Eighteen to twenty weeks

Answer: d. During the eighteenth to twentieth weeks' gestation the genders of the fetuses can be accurately determined on an abdominal ultrasound.

5. What is the most important thing for the obstetrician to follow in the third trimester in a twin gestation?
    a. Maternal weight gain
    b. Cervical dilatation status
    c. Maternal peripheral edema
    d. Maternal blood sugars

Answer: b. The most important thing to follow during the third trimester is the cervical dilatation status as this is an indicator of the possibility of a preterm birth.

6. Why is it more likely for twins to remain in the hospital longer after birth when compared to singleton babies?
   a. They have a greater chance of neonatal infections
   b. They have more feeding difficulties
   c. They are smaller than singleton babies
   d. They have more complications related to being preterm

Answer: d. Twins are more likely to be preterm at birth and will spend more time in the neonatal intensive care unit with complications related to being preterm.

7. Which complication of pregnancy is more likely to occur in the third trimester of a twin pregnancy when compared to a singleton pregnancy?
   a. Group B strep colonization
   b. Gestational hypertension
   c. Chorioamnionitis
   d. Placental insufficiency

Answer: b. Gestational hypertension is one complication of the third trimester that tends to occur more likely in women carrying twins when compared to a singleton pregnancy.

8. Why might a woman carrying twins have difficulty walking in the third trimester of pregnancy?
   a. The uterus impairs the woman's full ability to take a deep breath
   b. The uterus is so heavy that the woman is clumsier than if she were carrying one baby
   c. There is a greater chance of separation of the pubic symphysis in a twin pregnancy
   d. The woman will have more peripheral edema with a twin pregnancy

Answer: c. The larger uterus in a twin pregnancy will have a greater chance of causing separation of the pubic symphysis, which will make walking more difficult.

9. What is the biggest complication of having a twin-twin transfusion syndrome?
   a. Both babies have a higher chance of being anemic.
   b. One baby will get too much blood while the other baby will get too little blood.
   c. One baby will be bigger than the other.
   d. One baby will survive while the other baby will die.

Answer: b. Twin-twin transfusion syndrome is a serious complication in which one twin gets too much blood and one twin gets too little blood. It does not necessarily cause the death of either twin if managed appropriately.

10. Why is a fraternal twin gestation safer than having an identical twin gestation?
    a. The fraternal twins will be less likely to be born preterm.
    b. The fraternal twins will have fewer respiratory complications than identical twins.
    c. Fraternal twins don't have problems related to twin-twin transfusion syndrome.
    d. Fraternal twins tend to be much larger at birth than identical twins.

Answer: c. Fraternal twins have their own placenta, their own umbilical cord, and their own amniotic sac so there isn't the problem with twin-twin transfusion syndrome that can complicate an identical twin pregnancy.

Chapter 11: Spontaneous Abortions and Fetal Death

A spontaneous abortion is, by definition, a loss of pregnancy that occurs less than twenty weeks' gestation in the absence of any medical or surgical intervention, while a fetal death or fetal demise is a pregnancy loss that occurs any time after twenty weeks' gestation. In general, there are different factors that play into these types of pregnancy losses, which will be discussed as part of this chapter.

Spontaneous Abortion

There are several medical and non-medical terms used to describe a spontaneous abortion, including "spontaneous pregnancy loss", "miscarriage", or "early pregnancy failure". These terms tend to be more acceptable than using the word "abortion", which carries many negative connotations in today's society.

When evaluating a woman with a possible early pregnancy loss, a serum HCG level should be obtained. A single HCG value isn't as helpful as having two serial HCG levels that can be compared. In early pregnancy, there should be a doubling of the HCG level every forty-eight to seventy-two hours. If this doesn't happen, an early pregnancy loss should be suspected. If an ultrasound is obtained showing an empty uterus and the HCG level in a single reading is more than one thousand eight hundred mIU per milliliter, the index of suspicion for an ectopic pregnancy should be high and requires further evaluation.

A transvaginal ultrasound needs to be done for any suspected incomplete abortion to identify any retained products of conception. If retained products of conception are found, the woman may be followed with expectant management. There is an eighty-two to ninety-six percent success rate for a completed spontaneous abortion even without any intervention. When misoprostol or Cytotec is used for women who have suffered a missed spontaneous abortion, the pill should be given intravaginally instead of orally to open the cervix and trigger uterine contractions that will expel the products of conception.

Women who are Rh-negative should have a fifty-microgram dose of Rhogam, which is Rh immune globulin, to prevent sensitization at the time of the pregnancy loss. As these patients often have psychological reactions to their loss, the physician must be aware of these reactions and should be prepared to provide emotional support.

In a complete abortion, all the products of conception pass spontaneously without any medical or surgical intervention, while an incomplete abortion involves the partial passage of the products of conception with some tissues remaining in the uterus. An inevitable abortion involves the opening of the cervix in the absence of expulsion of the products of conception. In a missed abortion, there is evidence of a fetal demise, but the uterus does not show signs of eliminating the pregnancy products of conception. Recurrent spontaneous abortion refers to a woman who has at least three consecutive pregnancy losses in the first trimester. A septic abortion is any spontaneous pregnancy loss that is complicated by some type of uterine infectious process. A threatened abortion refers to a pregnancy prior to twenty weeks' gestation that is at a risk for a spontaneous abortion because of vaginal bleeding.

About a fifth of all women in pregnancy will have some type of vaginal bleeding prior to twenty weeks' gestation and about half of these will suffer a pregnancy loss. Up to twenty percent of pregnancies that are proven by a positive urine HCG evaluation will be lost. Women who have blood testing showing quantitative HCG levels over time will have a pregnancy loss that is as high as thirty-one percent. Even so, most miscarriages occur so early in gestation that the woman never knows she was pregnant.

A threatened abortion or vaginal bleeding in the context of a confirmed pregnancy is a common first trimester pregnancy complication. A full history and physical examination should take place in these settings to identify any possible cause of the threatened abortion. Lab tests should include a KOH prep of any vaginal discharge, a vaginal wet prep evaluation, a complete blood count, blood typing to include Rh testing, and quantitative serum HCG testing. High risk patients should have gonorrhea and chlamydia testing.

Ultrasound is critical to the diagnosis of a threatened abortion. If a transvaginal ultrasound is performed and reveals an empty uterus, this must be weighed against the serum HCG level. If the HCG level is greater than one thousand eight hundred mIU per milliliter, further evaluation for an ectopic pregnancy must be undertaken. If a transabdominal ultrasound is used and if the quantitative HCG level is higher than three thousand five hundred mIU per ml, an ectopic pregnancy should be considered if no pregnancy can be found in the uterus. An ectopic pregnancy can explain this finding as can a completed abortion in which the HCG level hasn't yet returned to normal. If a fetal heartbeat can be found on ultrasound in a threatened abortion, the risk of miscarriage drops from about fifty percent to about three percent.

The differential diagnoses to be considered when vaginal bleeding occurs in the first trimester include cervical friability, cervical cancer, trauma to the vagina or cervix, cervical polyps, ectopic pregnancy, idiopathic bleeding in a normal pregnancy, vaginal infection, cervicitis, molar pregnancy, spontaneous abortion, and sub-chorionic hemorrhage.

When the clinical examination shows a dilated cervix, the miscarriage becomes inevitable. However, an open cervix does not differentiate a completed miscarriage versus an incomplete miscarriage. This requires the use of a transvaginal ultrasonography, which is very reliable in identifying products of conception in the uterus. Transvaginal ultrasonography is also invaluable in identifying a missed spontaneous abortion.

Risk Factors and Etiology for a Spontaneous Abortion

The major cause of a spontaneous abortion is a chromosomal abnormality in the fetus. In one study, it was determined that major chromosomal abnormalities could be found in forty-nine percent of spontaneous abortions. The most common abnormality seen was an autosomal trisomy condition, which was seen in fifty-two percent of cases. Polyploidy accounted for twenty-one percent of cases, while monosomy X accounted for thirteen percent.

Most of the abnormalities were random events, such as a paternal or maternal defect in gametogenesis, nondisjunction of a chromosome, or dispermy. Structural chromosomal abnormalities of single chromosomes were found in six percent of cases and about half of these were inherited abnormalities.

In about four to six percent of recurrent spontaneous abortion cases, inherited chromosomal abnormalities have been found to be the cause of the recurrent losses.

There are multiple risk factors that go into a spontaneous pregnancy loss in the first trimester. It should be noted that things like stress, sexual intercourse, and marijuana use do not increase the risk of early pregnancy losses. Things that do increase the early pregnancy loss risk include advanced maternal age, use of alcohol, having inhalational anesthesia, drinking large amounts of caffeine, having chronic maternal diseases like poorly controlled diabetes mellitus, antiphospholipid antibody syndrome, celiac disease, and autoimmune diseases. Cigarette smoking also increases the risk of miscarriage. Women who use cocaine or have an intrauterine device will have a higher risk of miscarriage and any woman who conceives within three months of a previous pregnancy will have a higher rate of miscarriage.

The presence of several maternal infections will increase the risk of miscarriage including herpes simplex virus infections, bacterial vaginosis, mycoplasmosis, listeriosis, chlamydial infections, HIV disease, rubella, gonorrhea, malaria, parvovirus B19, and cytomegalovirus infections. Medications that can cause miscarriages include misoprostol (Cytotec), retinoids, NSAID medications, and methotrexate. A woman with many past elective abortions has an increased risk of miscarriage and having a previous pregnancy loss also increases the risk of a subsequent pregnancy loss. Toxic exposures to organic solvents, heavy metals, polyurethane, carbon disulfide, ethylene glycol, lead, and arsenic can increase the miscarriage risk. Certain uterine anomalies like fibroid tumors, adhesions, and abnormally-shaped uteruses can cause a higher than normal risk of a spontaneous abortion.

Treatment of Spontaneous Abortions

The major treatment intervention in the management of spontaneous abortions is the dilatation and curettage, which can remove any retained products of conception. Some surgeons opt for a manual vacuum aspiration of the contents of the uterus. In the past, it was felt to be urgent to remove the products of conception because of an increased risk for infection and coagulation disorders if the uterine contents weren't emptied. However, recent research indicates that expectant waiting is another good option that doesn't threaten the physical health of the mother.

Unstable patients or patients with septic abortions need to have urgent surgical evacuation of the contents of the uterus. In the absence of these things, the patient may make the decision as to whether to wait for a spontaneous loss or to have some type of surgical intervention.

In women who present after a completed abortion at home, an ultrasound will show an empty uterus and the tissue she brings in will be evaluated to ensure they are products of conception. If this cannot be proven, an ectopic pregnancy must be looked for.

As mentioned, there are many ways to manage threatened and incomplete miscarriages. Expectant management is successful in up to ninety-six percent of cases. Most patients who underwent surgical intervention were followed by expectant management for a couple of weeks before a surgical intervention was undertaken. Medical treatment with misoprostol or mifepristone doesn't seem to decrease the chances of having to have a surgical intervention. On average, it takes nine days from the onset of bleeding to the completion of the miscarriage.

Women who have missed miscarriages can be followed expectantly but the success rate is only about sixteen to seventy-six percent. Medical therapy for missed miscarriages has a high rate of success in completing a missed miscarriage. Misoprostol given to a woman with retained products of conception resulted in a completed abortion eighty percent of the time. The dose is eight hundred mcg of misoprostol given intravaginally twice, four hours apart. The side effect of diarrhea is much less likely to occur if the medication is given by this route than by the oral route.

Psychological Issues after a Spontaneous Abortion

Doctors need to be cognizant of the psychological issues that affect women experiencing spontaneous abortions. Although the literature doesn't usually address this factor, it is believed that the outcome of a spontaneous abortion is more successful when the patient's psychological factors are considered. The doctor should be aware of the impact of a spontaneous abortion on couple, who often feel sadness, grief, anxiety, depression, and guilty feelings. The doctor's role is to provide objective data indicating that the clear majority of miscarriages are not related to anything the mother did or didn't do during the pregnancy.

Grief should be encouraged and allowed to happen. Doctors need to counsel the woman that she may become frustrated by a lack of understanding of the grief she is experiencing. Many family members and friends will ignore the topic of miscarriage or will minimize it, which often makes things worse. Patients with these frustrations may do well with clinic or hospital-based support groups, where the full range of their feelings can be discussed.

There is a high risk of psychiatric problems in the weeks or months after spontaneous abortion. Women who were found to be particularly prone to psychiatric difficulties after a pregnancy loss are those who have no other children and were carrying a wanted pregnancy at the time of their loss. With no treatment for these issues, most women will recover from their psychological difficulties within twelve weeks after the loss.

Things to keep in mind that should be covered in managing the psychological aspects of a pregnancy loss include acknowledging the guilt and making attempts to dispel it. The grief is legitimate, and the doctor can help the patients realize this. The level of grief should be quantified, and interventions given according to how severe the problem is. Patients will need advice as to how to tell the friends and family about the loss and there should be every attempt at including the patient's partner in the decision-making and grief process. Simply offering comfort and support in an empathetic way will be of significant help to these patients, who also need practical advice regarding how to prevent a miscarriage in the future if this can be accomplished.

Management of Fetal Demise

Fetal demise, by definition, is the loss of fetal heartbeat and fetal death any time after twenty weeks' gestation. It is often confirmed by ultrasound. Women told they have suffered a fetal demise should be offered a prompt termination of the pregnancy, even though some will not be ready for this. Some women want to be induced immediately, while others need hours or days before they can decide and so they can be more emotionally-prepared at the time of termination.

The fetus cannot be left in the uterus for longer than three to four weeks because the fibrinogen levels drop in the maternal circulation, leading to bleeding complications from a coagulopathy. In cases where one twin has died, and the other twin has lived, induction of labor is delayed for as long as is feasible to allow the living twin to mature before delivery.

Induction starts with pre-induction cervical ripening with prostaglandin E2 gel. This is followed using intravenous oxytocin. Women who've had a previous cesarean section should be watched extremely carefully during a vaginal birth after cesarean or VBAC situation as there can be the complication of a uterine rupture. Early fetal loss can be managed by inserting laminaria in the cervix to allow it to dilate and then performing a curettage or vacuum evacuation. If the fetal death is prior to twenty-eight weeks' gestation, misoprostol or prostaglandin E2 can be given orally or intravaginally to bring on labor as this is a time when oxytocin inductions are less successful.

The treatment that offers the best option for the shortest labor and delivery after a fetal demise involves giving mifepristone orally at two hundred milligrams by mouth. This is followed using misoprostol 400 mcg every four to six hours orally or intravaginally. Misoprostol alone can also be highly effective. Mechanical ripening of the cervix can be achieved using a Foley catheter. After the cervix opens, an oxytocin induction can be undertaken.

As there is no risk for danger to the fetus, pain control should be aggressively managed in these labors. Patients often do well with epidural anesthesia, intravenous morphine therapy, or hydromorphone therapy given using a patient-controlled pump.

The causes of fetal demise are not known in up to sixty percent of cases. When a cause can be clearly defined, the cause of the death can have fetal, placental, or maternal factors playing into the fetal loss. One study indicated that the placenta was the cause of death in two-thirds of fetal demise situations. This is especially true when the fetal loss happens at a late gestational age.

A major modifiable risk factor that plays into the loss of a fetus after twenty weeks is maternal obesity. Advanced maternal age and smoking in pregnancy play a lesser role. Other risk factors found were the presence of a small for gestational age infant and placental abruption. Lesser risk factors include preexisting diabetes and preexisting hypertension that carry over in the pregnancy.

Maternal factors that increase the risk of fetal demise include a pregnancy lasting longer than forty-two weeks, poorly controlled maternal diabetes, lupus, antiphospholipid syndrome, maternal infection, maternal gestational hypertension, preeclampsia/eclampsia, hemoglobinopathies in the mother, advanced maternal age, Rh sensitization, uterine rupture, maternal trauma, and inherited blood hypercoagulability states.

Fetal factors that affect fetal demise include having a multiple gestation pregnancy, intrauterine growth restriction, congenital anomaly, genetic defect, fetal infection from bacteria or viruses, and hydrops fetalis.

Placental factors that play into having a fetal demise include a cord accident, abruption of the placenta, premature rupture of the membranes, vasa previa, fetomaternal hemorrhage, and placental insufficiency. Placental insufficiency is the most common cause of fetal demise after forty weeks' gestation.

Epidemiological factors that weakly predict the presence of fetal demise include being African-American, having an advanced maternal age, having a history of fetal demise, having maternal infertility in the past, having a small for gestational age fetus, being obese in pregnancy, and being of older paternal age.

Diagnosis of Fetal Demise

The time after a fetal demise is tumultuous for the family and the doctors who care for them. In this stressful period, it is the doctor's and nurse's jobs to stay in tune to the clues of grief, depression, anxiety, guilt, and other symptoms seen after a fetal demise. Grief packets should be readily available to give to patients who may need to read information previously provided that they likely forgot or failed to assimilate.

Folders and containers should be given to the family, in which they can place footprints, hand prints, locks of hair, photos, and other keepsakes. Information regarding support groups should be included in these packets for the patient and her spouse to call and arrange meetings with. Spiritual support should be offered to all families, based on their religious affiliation.

Experts don't agree on what testing should be done to evaluate a fetal demise. Up to sixty percent of stillbirths have no known etiology, even with a thorough workup. Even so, attempts should be made to find a cause as this can have an impact on future pregnancy plans and interventions that might help prevent another fetal loss. Obvious causes of fetal demise that require little ongoing evaluation include cord accidents, prolapsed cord, knot in the cord, entanglement of the cord, or a tight nuchal cord. Anencephaly or the presence of a previously known lethal chromosomal pattern in the fetus are other causes of fetal demise. If abruption was the cause of fetal demise, toxicology can be done, and the platelet count should be evaluated for thrombophilia.

The fetal autopsy is the most important part of the workup of fetal demise. If the parents don't want an autopsy, a full-body MRI scan can be undertaken. The membranes and placenta need to be evaluated for abnormalities and culturing. Amniotic fluid should be saved for karyotyping or a piece of fetal tissue can be harvested. Karyotyping should be undertaken if the fetus does not look normal because of abnormal facies, intrauterine growth restriction, or fetal hydrops. Multiple pregnancy losses should have karyotyping done on the deceased fetus. The parent's genetic makeup may also be necessary to identify any problems that will portend a future fetal demise.

Key Takeaways

- Spontaneous abortions happen prior to the twentieth week of gestation.
- A fetal demise happens after the twentieth week of gestation.
- Most pregnancy losses before term happen before the mother knows she's pregnant.
- Fetal demise can have maternal factors, placental factors, or fetal factors.
- Autopsies don't have to be done on every case of fetal demise but can help identify problems that may avert a repeat fetal demise in the subsequent pregnancies.

Quiz

1. What is the usual first sign that a woman is having a threatened spontaneous abortion?
   a. Low grade fever
   b. Vaginal bleeding
   c. Open cervix
   d. Lack of fetal heartbeat

Answer: b. Usually the first finding in a threatened spontaneous abortion is vaginal bleeding.

2. What is the main identifying feature in an inevitable miscarriage?
   a. Low HCG levels on a serum blood test
   b. Ultrasound showing the absence of a fetal heartbeat
   c. Opening the cervical os
   d. Maternal fever of up to 101.5 degrees Fahrenheit.

Answer: c. Once the cervical os is opened, the miscarriage is inevitable.

3. Which is the most common presentation in a missed abortion?
   a. Vaginal bleeding
   b. Fever
   c. Coagulopathy of undetermined origin
   d. Diminishing signs of pregnancy

Answer: d. A missed abortion means that the embryo or fetus has died but remains in the uterus. There may be no bleeding and there is no cramping. The only symptom may be a lack of pregnancy symptoms that were present before the fetal loss.

4. What percentage of pregnancies (documented and undocumented by a home pregnancy test) go on to miscarry in the first trimester?
   a. About ten percent
   b. About twenty percent
   c. About thirty percent
   d. About forty percent

Answer: c. Approximately thirty percent of all fertilized eggs and embryos that make enough HCG to be detected in the blood or urine eventually resorb and miscarry in the third trimester.

5. The woman has a mild placental abruption at 32-weeks' gestation. She is Rh-negative. The placental abruption clots spontaneously and the pregnancy is allowed to continue. Without medical intervention in this case, what is the most serious complication of this pregnancy?
   a. Fetal demise from Rh sensitivity in the mother
   b. Small for gestational age infant
   c. Fetal developmental delay
   d. Chorioamnionitis later in pregnancy

Answer: a. The most serious complication of a placental abruption in an Rh-negative mother is the mixing of maternal and fetal blood, causing fetal demise from Rh sensitization in the mother.

6. You are managing the care of a 32-year-old woman who has had an incomplete spontaneous abortion at 9 weeks' gestation. She wants to have the process over with and doesn't want the products of conception expelled as soon as possible. What medical therapy can you give her?
   a. Dilatation and curettage
   b. Misoprostol intravaginally
   c. Oxytocin intravenously
   d. Laminaria insertion

Answer: b. Misoprostol can be given intravaginally. It will help open the cervix and stimulate contractions and cramping that will expel the products of conception. Oxytocin will be ineffective at this point in the pregnancy and the other choices are not considered medical interventions

7. You are evaluating a woman who is being evaluated three-week visit after having a spontaneous abortion at 9 weeks' gestation, complicated by the need for a dilatation and curettage. What aspect of her care needs to be addressed the most?
   a. The provision of Rhogam
   b. Birth control option discussion
   c. Grief and loss issues
   d. Endometritis evaluation

Answer: c. At three weeks following the D and C, the chances of endometritis are remote. Rhogam should have already been given at the time of the procedure. Birth control options are much less of a priority than issues around grief and loss.

8. A fetus has suffered a fetal demise at 41 weeks' gestation. Statistically, what is the most common cause of fetal demise at this gestational age?
   a. Chromosomal abnormalities
   b. Maternal smoking history
   c. Placental insufficiency
   d. Chorioamnionitis

Answer: c. At 41 to 42 weeks' gestation, the most common cause of fetal demise is placental insufficiency as the placenta has aged so much that it cannot provide adequate amounts of nutrients and oxygen to the fetus.

9. You are counseling a woman who has just had a completed miscarriage in her 10th week of gestation. This is the third time in a row that this has happened in the first trimester to this woman. What should she be evaluated for?
   a. Luteal phase defect
   b. Fetal karyotype for inherited chromosome abnormalities
   c. Cervical swab for HPV infection
   d. Incompetent cervix

Answer: b. As all the woman's miscarriages are in the first trimester, they are not likely to be due to an incompetent cervix. A luteal phase defect will be problematic in extremely early pregnancy losses. HPV infections do not cause recurrent miscarriages but abnormalities in the fetal karyotype or parental karyotypes might point to a specific chromosomal abnormality causing the pregnancy losses.

10. A 28-weeks' gestation pregnancy with an average-sized, active infant is found to be complicated by oligohydramnios. The mother presents to the hospital because of a lack of fetal movement. The fetus has no heartbeat on ultrasound. Statistically, what is the most probable cause of this fetal demise?
    a. Fetal birth defect involving the kidneys
    b. Lack of fetal lung maturity
    c. Rh sensitization with fetal hydrops
    d. Umbilical cord accident

Answer: d. In a pregnancy near term with oligohydramnios, the cord has very little space in which to float freely. This increases the likelihood of the problem of a cord accident. The other choices are not complications of oligohydramnios that lead to fetal demise in utero.

Chapter 12: Contraception and Sterilization

After the birth of an infant, many couples want to resume sexual intercourse but without the risk of becoming pregnant. Other women are simply not willing to become mothers and want to have something that will prevent an unwanted pregnancy. This chapter evaluates the various choices available to a sexually active couple not wanting to conceive a child.

Intrauterine Contraception

The use of intrauterine contraception has gone in and out of favor over the past few decades. There are now two several types of intrauterine devices that will prevent pregnancy without the need to remember to take a pill every day or put a condom on prior to sexual intercourse.

The Copper T Intrauterine Device or IUD is a small plastic and metal device that is shaped like the letter "T". The doctor inserts the IUD inside the uterus. The IUD changes the milieu of the inner lining of the uterus so that embryos are unable to attach to the uterus. It can be inserted during an in an office procedure and will prevent pregnancies for up to ten years. The typical use failure rate is less than one percent, making it a very effective way to prevent pregnancy in women who want long-term pregnancy prevention.

Figure 12 shows what an IUD looks like:

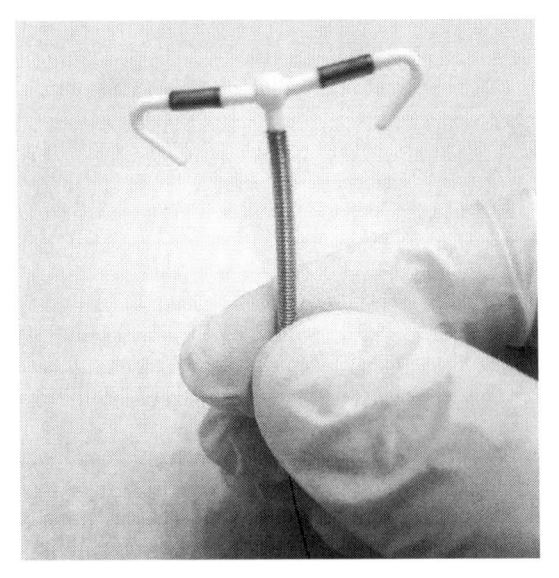

Figure 12

The levonorgestrel intrauterine system or LNG IUD is another copper T IUD that is inserted into the uterus by the doctor in an office visit. It elutes small amounts of progestin each day, which makes the lining of the uterus even more inhospitable for the implantation of a fertilized egg than a simple copper T device. Progestin also alters the vaginal and cervical mucus so that sperm cells have a more tough time getting into the cervix for fertilization.

Hormonal Methods of Birth Control

Young women often opt for a hormonal method of birth control. Hormones usually involve some element of estrogen and progesterone—both of which override the ovaries production of these hormones, inducing a quiescent state that has no eggs released. Some women prefer getting their hormonal birth control in pill forms, while others prefer an implant, a patch, or IUD.

The implant or Norplant is a rod-like device that is inserted under the skin of the woman's arm in an office outpatient procedure. The rod releases a steady state of progestin into the woman's body for up to three years. The failure rate of the implant is about 0.05 percent. The advantage of this form of birth control is there is nothing to remember until the three years are up. The main disadvantage is that the rods may be seen underneath the skin in thin women and they are sometimes extremely difficult to remove after they've scarred into the body during the three years they were implanted.

There is an injectable birth control method that involves seeing the doctor every three months and receiving an injection of long-acting progesterone. The most popular shot of this type is the Depo-Provera shot. Many women like it because it tends to eliminate periods while the injection is actively working in the body. It is not a good birth control method for obese women as weight gain can be a side effect. The woman also needs to return every three months to have the best effectiveness. The failure rate is about six percent.

Combined oral contraceptive pills are what most women refer to as the birth control pill. This is a pill that is taken at the same time of the day every day of the week. The pills come in a pack of twenty-one or twenty-eight pills. Three weeks of the pills will contain some form of estrogen and progestin, while the fourth week of the pills contains no active hormones. It triggers a period every three weeks with small amounts of bleeding while the active pills are taken.

Because these types of birth control pills contain estrogen, they cannot be taken by women who are older than thirty-five years of age and women who smoke as they raise the risk of stroke and coronary artery disease. Women with breast cancer and blood clots may also want to find some other form of birth control as there is a risk of breast cancer and deep vein thromboses of the leg while the woman takes the pill.

The progestin only pill or mini-pill is also taken every day at the same time of the day. It contains only progestins that make the hormonal milieu of the uterine lining not receptive for implantation should an egg be fertilized. It is good for breastfeeding women as it contains no estrogen. Women with side effects from estrogen or who have risk factors that preclude estrogen use are good candidates for this type of pill. The failure rate is about the same as with the combination pill at around nine percent.

The skin patch is another hormonal method of birth control, containing estrogen and progestin. The patch is placed on the buttocks, the lower abdomen, or the upper body of the woman but cannot be placed on the breasts. A patch is placed on the skin every week for three weeks and then, during the fourth week, the patch is removed and the woman has her period. The typical use failure rate of this type of contraception is nine percent, although obese women have a higher failure rate using the patch.

There is a hormonal vaginal contraceptive ring. The ring releases progestins and estrogen directly into the vagina by leaching out of the vaginal ring. The ring is worn inside the vagina for three weeks and is taken out for the week when the period is expected. A new ring is then replaced after the period is over with. The typical use failure rate is about nine percent.

Emergency Contraception

Emergency contraception uses high dose hormones that are given after a woman fears she has become pregnant after unprotected sex. It is given to a woman after a rape situation or after she has had sex using a failed barrier method. If the pill has been given within 72 hours after intercourse, it can prevent pregnancies with a failure rate of about fifteen to twenty-five percent.

Women can also choose to have the Copper T IUD Inserted as a form of emergency birth control that doesn't involve hormones. The IUD needs to be inserted within five days of having unprotected sex. Combination oral contraceptives containing ethynyl estradiol and norgestrel can be given after unprotected sex. Two doses of this type of pill are taken twelve hours a part beginning before seventy-two hours have passed since the time of intercourse. The progestin-only oral contraceptive pill, which contains levonorgestrel, can be used for emergency contraception. Two doses are given twelve hours apart beginning before seventy-two hours have passed since the time of intercourse.

Plan B is a pill specifically designed for use as emergency contraception. It contains 1.5 milligrams of levonorgestrel at one time or half that amount given twice at twelve hours apart. It costs about $22 and can be used sporadically in woman who have failed their usual backup method. The sooner these hormonal methods are given after intercourse, the better they are at preventing a pregnancy. A time frame of about seventy-two hours after unprotected sex is considered adequate to prevent pregnancy when using plan B.

Barrier Methods

There are several barrier methods that have the advantage of providing better protection against sexually transmitted diseases when compared to hormonal birth control methods. The diaphragm or cervical cap is a rubber-like device that can be placed over the cervix to cover the external os of the cervix so sperm cannot get into the uterus. The diaphragm is bigger and is shaped like a soft-bottom cup. It is often used with spermicides, which improve adhesion of the diaphragm to the cervix and help kill sperm cells as they pass near the cervix. The cervical cap is shaped like the diaphragm but is much smaller and fits directly over the cervix. The typical use failure rate is twelve percent.

The male condom is a commonly used form of birth control. It is usually made from latex but can be made from other synthetic substances. They make "natural" condoms from lambskin. While these natural condoms will prevent pregnancy, they don't protect a person from STDs, including HIV disease. The typical use failure rate of the male condom is eighteen percent. Their main disadvantage is that they can only be used once and must be used with a water-based lubricant because oil-based lubricants such as baby oil, massage oils, lotions, or petrolatum jelly will weaken a latex condom.

The female condom is worn by the woman to prevent sperm from entering the cervix. It comes from a regular pharmacy and has lubricant in the packaging. It is inserted in the female vagina up to eight hours prior to having sex. It can prevent some sexually transmitted diseases but has a typical use failure rate of twenty-one percent.

Spermicides alone can be protective against a pregnancy. They come in several different forms, including gels, foams, films, suppositories, creams, or tablets. Spermicides are placed into the vagina within an hour of an anticipated intercourse and cannot be washed out or removed for six to eight hours after sex. Spermicides are most effective when used along with a male condom, a female condom, a diaphragm, or a cervical cap. The failure rate when used alone is about twenty-eight percent.

Fertility Awareness Methods of Contraception

This method of contraception is nothing more than teaching the woman to recognize what is going on during her monthly cycles. The biggest disadvantage is that it depends on the woman having normal and regular menstrual cycles. The woman learns her fertility pattern by taking basal body temperature readings and evaluating her cervical mucus. She learns to recognize those days when she is most likely to get pregnant and avoids having sexual relations or decides to use a barrier method on those days. The typical use failure rate of this method of birth control is twenty-four percent.

Tubal Ligation

The tubal ligation is a birth control method that is designed to offer the woman permanent contraception, even though it is technically possible to reverse this surgical procedure when a pregnancy is again desired. It should be known that, while this is a reversible procedure, the tube may not be as patent after surgical repair and there will be a higher than normal risk of an ectopic pregnancy and there may not be a complete return to normal fertility after reversal.

Prior to doing a tubal ligation, the woman should have a urine HCG test to qualitatively identify those situations in which the woman is already pregnant before having her tubal ligation. The test should be done on the day of the tubal ligation surgery. If the test is negative during the luteal phase of the menstrual cycle, the limitations of the test make it nearly impossible to know for sure if the woman is pregnant at the time of her surgery. For this reason, it is better to do a serum HCG qualitative test and do the tubal ligation in the first half of the woman's cycle before she ovulates. The woman should have had a normal pap test within six months of the surgery and should have preoperative lab testing that includes screening for gonorrhea and chlamydia, a hemoglobin/hematocrit, and a urinalysis. If the woman tests positive for either gonorrhea or chlamydia, the procedure should be delayed until the infection has abated.

There are several therapeutic approaches to the surgery that sterilizes the female reproductive tract. Laparoscopy, hysteroscopy, microlaparoscopy, minilaparotomy, laparotomy (during a Cesarean section), mini-laparotomy, and vaginal approaches have all been used to disrupt the patency of the fallopian tubes. The most commonly used approach throughout the world is the minilaparotomy; however, the laparoscopy is the most widely used technique for doing a tubal ligation in the US. Procedures involving the use of hysteroscopy are gaining in popularity as more doctors are learning the technique.

Postpartum women who've had a vaginal delivery can have a simple laparoscopic procedure that can be done a day or two after delivery.

The puerperal tubal ligation is relatively simple. The patient has an incision placed just under the umbilicus, which is where the top of the uterine fundus is located after birth. The fallopian tubes are easily visualized through this mini-incision and can be ligated. A bilateral tubal ligation can also simply be done as a tack-on procedure after an uncomplicated cesarean section. Any delay of doing the tubal ligation after childbirth for more than a few days makes the mini-laparotomy procedure not as successful so the procedure might need to be done by means of laparoscopy or hysteroscopy.

The minilaparotomy is basically the same as a laparotomy but involves making an incision shorter than two inches in the suprapubic area of the woman's abdomen. The incision is just beneath the umbilicus if the woman is within 48 hours from given birth.

Laparoscopy can be used in a woman at any point in her childbearing years. Several small cuts are placed to allow for trocars to enter the pelvis and abdomen. The trocars, a camera, and lights are used with surgical tools that can identify the fallopian tubes, tie them off, and ligate a section of the tube on either side of the uterus. The laparoscopy has benefits as the recovery time is less, but it has complications, especially with obese individuals. About half of all complications come from a problem with the entry of the laparoscope. The success rate of a laparoscopic sterilization is about ninety-nine percent, while the success rate of a hysteroscopic tubal ligation is only about eighty eight percent on the first attempt.

Key Takeaways

- Most contraceptive methods are directly related to altering some aspect of the female reproductive cycle. These methods have the best success rate when used correctly.
- Barrier methods exist for both the man and the woman in the form of the diaphragm, the cervical cap, the female condom, and the male condom. These have lesser rates of contraceptive success.
- Tubal ligation in women is a permanent form of sterilization that is done in an operating room. It is designed to be permanent but can technically be reversed with varying degrees of successfulness.

Quiz

1. You are counseling a nursing mother who has a three-month old infant. What type of birth control method can you recommend that will be the most effective in preventing a pregnancy?
    a. Fertility-based contraceptive techniques
    b. Breastfeeding to reduce fertility
    c. Progestin-only birth control pill
    d. Combination birth control pill

Answer: c. Women who are breastfeeding and want a hormonal birth control option that will be very effective can take a progestin-only birth control pill, which is also called the mini-pill.

2. The woman you are counseling had unprotected intercourse five days ago and wants something to prevent a pregnancy. What can you recommend for her?
    a. Plan B
    b. Single dose of ethynyl estradiol and norgestrel
    c. Combination birth control pills taken for the next five days at once per day
    d. Insertion of a copper T IUD

Answer: d. Any hormonal method of emergency contraception tends only to be effective if used within seventy-two hours after intercourse. The Copper T IUD can be used if placed within five days of unprotected intercourse.

3. Why would you recommend that a 17-year-old girl using Norplant as a form of birth control also use condoms during sexual intercourse?
    a. The Norplant device has a modestly high failure rate, so condoms can improve its effectiveness.
    b. Norplant doesn't protect against STDs, so this high-risk woman should also use condoms.
    c. Norplant takes a couple of months to become effective, so condoms are recommended.
    d. Norplant wears off after three months so it's a good idea to get into the habit of using condoms in case the follow up visits don't happen on schedule.

Answer: b. Norplant is extremely effective alone in preventing pregnancy, but it does not protect against STDs. For this reason, condoms should be recommended in high-risk women and teens.

4. A woman with a history of a deep vein thrombosis in her leg five years ago seeks birth control that will be effective and easy to remember. What birth control method might you suggest?
    a. Copper T IUD
    b. Ethynyl estradiol/norgestrel pills
    c. Diaphragm
    d. Cervical cap

Answer: a. This woman is at a high risk of getting another DVT and should be offered a birth control option with a low failure rate. She can't take any estrogen-containing birth control pill; however, the copper T IUD is highly effective, easy to remember, and won't adversely affect her blood clotting risk.

5. You are counseling a 14-year-old woman about birth control. She desires the Depo-Provera shot to be given every three months. What major side effect should you explain to her before giving her the shot?
    a. Heavy vaginal bleeding
    b. Weight gain
    c. Insulin resistance
    d. Vaginal dryness

Answer: b. The major side effect of Depo-Provera is weight gain. Teens especially may decide not to follow through with tri-monthly injections if they find it is causing them to gain weight, so they need to be informed about this side effect in advance.

6. What testing is imperative to do for a woman who is scheduled to have a tubal ligation within the next twenty-four hours?
    a. Ultrasound of the pelvis
    b. Serum progesterone level
    c. Serum HCG level
    d. Serum LH level

Answer: c. A serum HCG level should be done to rule out a pregnancy before doing the tubal ligation. Ideally, the testing should be done after a menstrual period but before ovulation has taken place.

7. What medical risk does a woman face if she chooses to have a reversal of her tubal ligation?
    a. Primary ovarian failure
    b. Pelvic inflammatory disease
    c. Polycystic ovarian disease
    d. Ectopic pregnancy

Answer: d. Because it is not possible to have completely smooth fallopian tube walls after repair of a previous tubal ligation, the egg or embryo can get hung up in the fallopian tube, resulting in an ectopic pregnancy.

8. What is the typical use failure rate of the combination birth control pill?
    a. One percent
    b. Five percent
    c. Nine percent
    d. Twenty percent

Answer: c. The typical use failure rate of the combination birth control pill is about nine percent?

9. Which birth control method listed has the lowest typical use failure rate?
    a. Copper T IUD
    b. Mini-pill
    c. Depo-Provera injection
    d. Spermicidal jelly

Answer: a. The Copper T IUD has less than a one percent failure rate. The other choices have a nine percent, six percent, and twenty-eight percent failure rates, respectively.

10. What is the main requirement for the success of the fertility awareness method of birth control?
    a. The willingness to always use condoms
    b. The willingness to use Plan B on a regular basis
    c. Predictable menstrual cycles
    d. Monogamous relationship

Answer: c. Because fertility awareness methods require that a woman pay close attention to her fertility at any point in her cycle, the thing that is practically a requirement for its successfulness is the presence of predictable menstrual cycles.

Summary

This course was a discussion of the practice of obstetrics. While obstetrics is generally practiced by an obstetrician/gynecologist, many family practice physicians also engage in obstetrical practice. The course covered both normal obstetrical care and the care of obstetrical complications.

The first chapter covered the reproductive anatomy of adult women, including the external anatomy such as the vulva, the labia majora, and the clitoris. It also covered the internal anatomy that cannot be seen, including the ovaries, the uterus, and the cervix.

In the second chapter of the course, the diagnosis of pregnancy was discussed. In modern times, pregnancy is diagnosed by a variety of methods, including blood levels of beta human chorionic gonadotropin, urine pregnancy tests, and ultrasonography. Even with modern technology, sometimes it just takes a good history and physical examination to diagnose a pregnancy.

The third chapter of the course was devoted to the physiological changes that occur in pregnancy. Pregnancy affects the cardiovascular system, the respiratory system, the gastrointestinal tract, the kidneys and ureters, the endocrine system, and the skin.

The fourth chapter discussed antepartum care of the normal pregnancy. Women tend to see the obstetrician sometime in the first trimester and are followed at routine visits throughout the pregnancy.

An extensive discussion of intrapartum care was discussed in the fifth chapter of the course. Women in labor and their fetuses require close observation during the labor process to make the process go as smoothly as possible without any intrapartum complications.

The sixth chapter of the course was a discussion of the postpartum period. Technically, the postpartum period starts when the placenta is delivered and ends at an arbitrary six-week checkup, although the woman will continue to undergo post-pregnancy changes for many months after giving birth. There can even be psychological changes that occur as late as twelve months after giving birth.

The seventh chapter of the course involved a discussion of medical conditions in pregnancy. Some pregnancies are high risk from the beginning because of a maternal health problem, such as hypertension or diabetes. Other pregnancies become complicated by the development of health problems unrelated to the reproductive system that are still impacted by the woman being pregnant.

The eighth chapter of the course was devoted to the various obstetrical complications that may occur. Most pregnancies are normal and result in full term and healthy babies, but others are complicated by external and internal factors.

Infections in pregnancy were also discussed. Most of the infections that affect a pregnancy are directly related to the female reproductive system; however, infections such as listeriosis have nothing to do with the reproductive system but still have serious consequences for the fetus or neonate.

The tenth chapter of the course was a discussion of twin pregnancies. Twin pregnancies happen often enough that most doctors who participate in obstetrical care will encounter many twin gestations in their practice.

The eleventh chapter of the course was a discussion of spontaneous abortions and fetal demise. Spontaneous abortions are miscarriages that happen prior to the twentieth week of pregnancy, while a fetal demise occurs at any time after the twentieth week gestation.

Finally, the last chapter of the book was a discussion of contraception in women as well as the sterilization process. Most women of reproductive age will need contraception if they are sexually active and don't desire to be pregnant. A woman who feels she is finished with the reproductive process may elect to have a tubal ligation, which is, for the most part, a permanent solution to getting pregnant.

Course Test Questions

1. In looking at a model of the female reproductive anatomy, where would you expect to find the bulk of the pubic hair?
    a. Mons pubis
    b. Labia minora
    c. Clitoris
    d. Labia majora

2. In an evaluation of the female vagina, you notice structures that are believed to be stretch enough to allow for the passage of the fetus in the second stage of labor. What are these called?
    a. Suspensory ligaments
    b. Rugae
    c. Hymen
    d. Erectile tissues

3. Where during an evaluation of a woman's external genitalia would you most likely find an erectile structure?
    a. Hymen
    b. Labia minora
    c. Clitoris
    d. Skene gland

4. Which structure in female reproductive anatomy can be found intact only when a young woman has not had the onset of menses?
    a. Clitoris
    b. Hymen
    c. Labia minora
    d. External os of the cervix

5. Which component of the female reproductive anatomy will change continuously throughout the month depending on the woman's hormone levels?
    a. Fallopian tubes
    b. Endometrium
    c. External cervical os
    d. Vaginal rugae

6. Approximately how many mature eggs does a woman's ovaries release as part of all the menstrual cycles she has during her lifetime?
    a. Fifty
    b. One hundred
    c. Three hundred
    d. One thousand

7. The ovaries are suspended in several ways. Which ligament can be referred to as the suspensory ligament of the ovaries?
   a. Broad ligament
   b. Ovarian ligament
   c. Mesovarium
   d. Infundibular pelvic ligament

8. When the ovaries are looked at under the microscope, what histological finding is most likely to be identified?
   a. Sheets of immature egg cells in columns
   b. Connective tissue bands supporting immature egg cell structures
   c. Cystic structures of varying sizes representing follicles of different ages
   d. Scar tissue islands representing sclerosed follicles

9. You are doing a gross inspection of several female uteruses. Which patient would likely have the smallest uterine weight in grams?
   a. A pre-adolescent female
   b. A nulligravida 25-year-old female
   c. A multigravida 30-year-old female
   d. A 70-year-old postmenopausal female

10. The doctor suspects that the woman is pregnant and does an abdominal exam. She can palpate the uterus as being below the pubic symphysis. What can be inferred based on this examination?
    a. The woman has an ectopic pregnancy.
    b. The woman is in her second trimester of pregnancy.
    c. The woman is less than twelve weeks' gestation.
    d. The woman probably has an inevitable spontaneous abortion.

11. In examining a woman who is believed to be pregnant, the doctor notices a positive Chadwick sign. What causes this sign in pregnancy?
    a. Venous congestion of the cervix
    b. Thinning of the cervix
    c. The presence of endometrial cells at the external os of the cervix
    d. The presence of a cervix much lower in the vaginal canal than is seen in non-pregnant females

12. The doctor is examining the cervix while doing a bimanual examination on a 29-year-old female and detects a positive Hegar sign. At what gestational age should this sign be noticeable for the first time?
    a. Four weeks' gestation
    b. Six weeks' gestation
    c. Eight weeks' gestation
    d. Twelve weeks' gestation

13. A newly pregnant woman has a serum HCG level of three hundred mIU per milliliter. In trying to decide if this is a false positive pregnancy test, what lab work can be done that will support the idea that the serum HCG level is a false positive test?
    a. A serum progesterone level
    b. A serum early pregnancy factor level
    c. A urine qualitative pregnancy test
    d. A repeat serum HCG level in two days

14. The ultrasound technician is attempting to evaluate the viability of a fetus by doing a transvaginal ultrasound looking for a fetal heartbeat. At what fetal pole size should the heartbeat first be detected?
    a. Two millimeters
    b. Five millimeters
    c. 50 millimeters
    d. One centimeter

15. The doctor is trying to establish that a pregnancy is viable early in the first trimester. At what progesterone level can she be relatively assured of the existence of a healthy pregnancy?
    a. Five nanograms per milliliter
    b. Twenty-five nanograms per milliliter
    c. Fifty nanograms per milliliter
    d. Seventy-five nanograms per milliliter

16. The technician is performing a transvaginal ultrasound on a woman believed to be newly pregnant. At what gestational age would the technician be able to see a fetal pole?
    a. Four to five weeks
    b. Five to six weeks
    c. Six to seven weeks
    d. Seven to eight weeks

17. Why is it a good idea to combine the technology of a transvaginal ultrasound along with HCG testing to identify a healthy pregnancy?
    a. Transvaginal ultrasounds are not very precise in identifying pregnancies before six weeks' gestation.
    b. The HCG level is better able to predict a healthy pregnancy when the ultrasound findings support the lab test.
    c. There are discriminatory levels that mean certain structures need to be present in a healthy pregnancy at certain HCG levels.
    d. The HCG alone cannot predict a healthy pregnancy.

18. Home pregnancy tests use a specific type of technology to detect a pregnancy. What type of testing is involved in these tests?
    a. Immunometric assay

b. Immunoradiometric assay
   c. Enzyme-linked immunosorbent assay
   d. Radiometric assay

19. The doctor is evaluating a woman regarding the cardiac changes seen in her pregnancy. Which statement about the heart changes in pregnancy is true?
    a. The stroke volume decreases
    b. The cardiac output increases
    c. The heart rate decreases
    d. The chances of arrhythmia are remote

20. The doctor performs a complete physical examination on a woman and finds that she has an enlarged thyroid gland and an elevated total thyroxine level in the second trimester of her pregnancy. What is the next thing that needs to be done to further evaluate this finding?
    a. Perform a thyroid gland biopsy
    b. Obtain a radionuclide thyroid scan
    c. Obtain a total triiodothyronine level
    d. Do nothing as this is a physiological response in pregnancy

21. What is the specific action of progesterone on the maternal respiratory status?
    a. It decreases the partial pressure of oxygen
    b. It decreases the oxygen saturation
    c. It decreases the respiratory rate
    d. It decreases the carbon dioxide level

22. What factors in the activities of a pregnant woman can cause an increase in kidney function?
    a. Lying on the left side
    b. Standing up
    c. Aerobically exercising
    d. Lying supine

23. What phenomenon explains the skin pigment changes seen in pregnancy?
    a. Increased risk of darkening of the skin from the sun
    b. Increased keratinization of the skin tissues
    c. Increased melanocyte stimulating hormone
    d. Increased progesterone level from the placenta

24. If a serum prolactin level is drawn from the blood of a woman at thirty-six weeks' gestation, what would be expected regarding the result?
    a. A normal serum prolactin level as the patient hasn't breastfed yet
    b. A two-fold increase in prolactin level
    c. A ten-fold increase in prolactin level

d. A one hundred-fold increase in prolactin level

25. Why is there frequently the finding of peripheral edema in an examination of a pregnant woman?
    a. A decrease in the glomerular filtration rate
    b. An increase in water and salt uptake by the kidneys
    c. A decrease in serum aldosterone level
    d. An increase in serum progesterone level

26. What gross physical finding can be noted in a woman's urinary tract system while she is pregnant?
    a. An enlargement of both kidneys
    b. A shrinkage of the bladder
    c. A widening of the ureters
    d. A foreshortening of the urethra

27. What is the primary cause of breast engorgement and tenderness among women who are in the early stages of pregnancy?
    a. Elevated progesterone levels
    b. Elevated HCG levels
    c. Elevated estradiol levels
    d. Elevated prolactin levels

28. Why is insulin resistance a natural part of the physiology of a pregnant woman?
    a. Increased estradiol levels
    b. Increased cortisol levels
    c. Increased HCG levels
    d. Increased alkaline phosphatase levels

29. When is it a good idea for a woman to schedule a pre-pregnancy gynecological visit?
    a. Only if she is older than thirty-five years of age
    b. Only if she suffers from infertility
    c. Only if she has an underlying medical problem before becoming pregnant
    d. Any time a woman wants to make sure she is healthy enough for a pregnancy

30. When in a woman's pregnancy is the maternal screening test for gestational diabetes performed?
    a. At the first prenatal visit
    b. Anytime sugar is found in the urine
    c. At twenty-four weeks
    d. At thirty-two weeks

31. Preterm labor can be defined as any labor that occurs before which gestational age?
    a. Twenty-eight weeks
    b. Thirty-two weeks

c. Thirty-five weeks
d. Thirty-seven weeks

32. What laboratory study is not tested as part of the triple screen?
    a. Fetal karyotype
    b. Human chorionic gonadotropin
    c. Alpha fetoprotein
    d. Conjugated estriol

33. When in a woman's pregnancy does an amniocentesis usually occur if this test is found to be necessary?
    a. Ten to twelve weeks
    b. Fourteen to sixteen weeks
    c. Eighteen to twenty weeks
    d. Twenty to twenty-two weeks

34. Pregnant women often get heartburn. Which recommendation could be given to her to help reduce this symptom?
    a. Take an antacid with every meal
    b. Avoid taking aspirin
    c. Elevate the head of the bed at night
    d. Eat a high protein diet

35. A woman asks you what she can do to avoid getting the Zika virus. What can she do to reduce her risk?
    a. Avoid unwashed vegetables
    b. Avoid processed lunchmeats
    c. Avoid travel to endemic countries
    d. Avoid intercourse with anyone other than her sexual partner

36. What is the best description of the four-dimensional ultrasound?
    a. It gives snapshots of the fetus's structures using sound waves
    b. It gives intricate detail of the fetus's inner organs
    c. It gives realistic pictures of the fetus's facial features
    d. It combines images of the fetus and evaluates fetal movements

37. A woman being seen in labor is six centimeters dilated and is experiencing a slowdown in the strength and frequency of her contractions. What first step can you do that will increase the rate of her contractions?
    a. Have her sit on the toilet
    b. Perform an amniotomy
    c. Add IV fluids to her treatment plan
    d. Give prostaglandin E2 gel to the cervix

38. Why shouldn't the obstetrician or family doctor do an amniotomy in the latent phase of labor in an HIV-infected mother?
    a. It will increase her bleeding risk.
    b. It increases the chance of getting chorioamnionitis.
    c. It tends not to increase the strength and frequency of her contractions.
    d. It increases the fetus's exposure to the HIV virus in utero.

39. The woman is being seen in the labor and delivery unit and is in the first stage of labor. What clinical finding warrants further investigation?
    a. A sudden gush of clear fluid from the vagina
    b. A maternal temperature of 99.0 degrees Fahrenheit
    c. Continuous abdominal pain
    d. Increased urinary frequency

40. The doctor believes that a woman in the second stage of labor needs an episiotomy. What is the main advantage of doing a mediolateral episiotomy?
    a. It is technically easier to do
    b. The blood loss is less
    c. There is less pain with this type of episiotomy
    d. There is no chance of extension into the rectum

41. The doctor is examining a pregnant woman at term before she goes into labor and suspects there will be shoulder dystocia. What things might lead the doctor to be prepared for this obstetrical complication?
    a. Previous baby weighing nine pounds
    b. Gestational diabetes
    c. Onset of labor at thirty-seven weeks
    d. Male gender of fetus

42. Why might the doctor choose to tell the laboring woman to wait on pushing in the second stage until there is bulging of the perineum?
    a. Pushing too early can lead to fetal distress
    b. Pushing late in the second stage provides less blood loss
    c. Pushing late in the second stage provides for more effective pushing
    d. The baby will be delivered just as quickly if she waits

43. What is the most common cause of bleeding in the third stage of labor?
    a. Retained placenta or placental fragments
    b. Uterine laceration
    c. Cervical laceration
    d. Full bladder

44. The doctor is managing a woman who has sustained a postpartum hemorrhage. What is the definition of a postpartum hemorrhage as it relates to this woman?
    a. She has lost blood after the delivery of the placenta

- b. She required blood transfusions after the delivery
- c. She lost more than 500 milliliters of blood in twenty-four hours
- d. She required intraoperative intervention to control bleeding

45. During the examination of the placenta after birth, a firm blood clot on the side of the placenta that had been attached to the uterine wall is visualized. What can this mean?
    - a. The patient has a cotyledon left in the placenta
    - b. The woman has normal clotting factors and doesn't have a bleeding disorder
    - c. She had an area of placental infarction near term
    - d. She had a partially abrupted placenta near term

46. A new mother is being evaluated prior to being discharged from the hospital after an uncomplicated vaginal delivery. If the mother and infant are stable, what is the accepted minimum amount of time the woman should be in the hospital before allowing her to go home?
    - a. Three hours
    - b. Six hours
    - c. Twelve hours
    - d. Forty-eight hours

47. A woman presents to the emergency room with the sudden onset of a red, tender breast and a fever. She is breastfeeding a two-week-old infant. How should this woman's problem be addressed?
    - a. Restrict breastfeeding to the normal breast until the infection resolves.
    - b. Instruct the woman to use hot compresses on the affected breast.
    - c. Provide the woman with an antibiotic that does not penetrate breast milk.
    - d. Provide the woman with an antibiotic that is safe when ingested by the newborn.

48. A 30-year old woman is being seen in the clinic. She is nursing her two-month-old infant and wants something for birth control. What is the most effective birth control method you can prescribe or recommend for her?
    - a. Diaphragm
    - b. Male condom
    - c. Mini-pill
    - d. Estradiol/Progestin pill

49. The patient is a 35-year-old woman who is breastfeeding and has clinical signs and symptoms of postpartum depression. What treatment can be given safely to her while she breastfeeds?
    - a. Nortriptyline
    - b. Amitriptyline

c. Fluoxetine
d. Electroconvulsive therapy

50. The patient in question has just had a vaginal delivery. At what time can you expect her uterus to shrink to its pre-pregnancy size?
    a. Two weeks
    b. Four weeks
    c. Six weeks
    d. It will never shrink to the pre-pregnancy size

51. A woman being seen by a visiting home nurse is one week postpartum and has symptoms of tearfulness and low mood that have not impacted her sleep, appetite, or her care of her newborn. The nurse can tell the woman these symptoms are likely to last for how long?
    a. Two weeks
    b. Six weeks
    c. Two months
    d. Six months

52. The husband of a postpartum woman calls to say his wife is hallucinating and has illogical thoughts. She is unable to care for her infant and he needs to do all the childcare. What advice should you give him?
    a. He should make an appointment for his wife to see a psychiatrist.
    b. He should start giving her an antipsychotic drug that you will provide for her.
    c. He needs to have her seen urgently in the emergency department.
    d. He needs to pick up a prescription for an antidepressant medication to give her.

53. In talking about postpartum depression with a woman who is having the symptoms of the disorder, what do you tell her the incidence is of this problem among postpartum women?
    a. One to two percent
    b. Four to six percent
    c. Ten to twenty percent
    d. Twenty to thirty percent

54. The doctor's job is to discuss birth control methods and contraception with all postpartum patients. At what point after the childbirth should this discussion take place under ideal circumstances?
    a. At the time of hospital discharge
    b. At two weeks' postpartum
    c. At the six-week postpartum visit

        d.   By the sixth postpartum month

55. A postpartum mother presents to the clinic with the complaint of constipation after having an unremarkable vaginal delivery without an episiotomy the week before. What can be recommended for her that will help this problem?
    a.   Bisacodyl suppositories
    b.   Fluids and increased fiber
    c.   Milk of Magnesia
    d.   Mylanta

56. A pregnant woman is in her third trimester and is found on examination to have a resting blood pressure of 165/100. What is the next test that should be done to evaluate this finding?
    a.   Electrocardiogram
    b.   Brachial ankle index
    c.   Urine dipstick for protein
    d.   Serum protein level

57. The woman being evaluated in the emergency department is 32-weeks' gestational age with a blood pressure reading of 155/95. The urinalysis shows 3+ protein in the urine. What can be given to her to prevent eclampsia?
    a.   IV nitroprusside
    b.   Oral labetalol
    c.   IV hydralazine
    d.   IV magnesium sulfate

58. The woman being seen in the hospital is a 32-year-old multiparous woman with preeclampsia. When can she be safely assured of having no neurological complication from this problem?
    a.   As soon as her blood pressure reaches below the 140/90 threshold
    b.   As soon as she delivers her infant
    c.   About three to four days after delivery
    d.   After receiving at least forty-eight hours of labetalol orally

59. The patient is a primiparous woman who is having routine prenatal care. As part of this care, when should she have a one-hour glucose tolerance test for gestational diabetes?
    a.   First prenatal visit
    b.   Twelve weeks' gestational age
    c.   Eighteen weeks' gestational age
    d.   Twenty-four weeks' gestational age

60. A woman with type 2 diabetes on metformin becomes pregnant and sees her primary care physician for management of her diabetes. How will her diabetes be managed during the pregnancy?
    a. She will remain on metformin but will monitor her blood sugars three times a day.
    b. She will stop the metformin and start a program of insulin therapy.
    c. She will stop the metformin and will begin a strict diet and exercise program for her diabetes.
    d. She will check blood sugars four times daily and will switch to Victoza (liraglutide)

61. A 30-year-old overweight female is in her first trimester of pregnancy and has a baseline history of hypertension. In managing her hypertension in pregnancy, what would a first line medication be for this?
    a. Labetalol
    b. Nifedipine
    c. Captopril
    d. Losartan

62. The doctor is caring for an infant who was born to a mother has known chronic hepatitis B. How is this handled?
    a. The infant is given the hepatitis B vaccine at two weeks of age.
    b. The infant is tested for the virus and, if negative, is given the hepatitis B vaccine.
    c. The infant is given the hepatitis B immune globulin.
    d. The infant is given the hepatitis B immune globulin and the hepatitis B vaccine on the day of birth.

63. The doctor is caring for an infant who was born to a mother who had an active gonorrhea infection at the time of a vaginal birth. How should the infant be treated?
    a. The infant is given oral systemic antibiotics against gonorrhea.
    b. A blood culture is obtained and the infant is treated if positive for gonorrhea.
    c. The infant is given erythromycin eye drops to protect against gonorrhea conjunctivitis.
    d. The infant is intravenous antibiotics against gonorrhea.

64. The doctor is caring for a pregnant woman who tested positive for HIV at the time of her first prenatal visit. For what reason is this test done on all pregnant women?
    a. Many pregnant women are high risk for HIV so they should be screened whenever they become pregnant.
    b. There will be a lot of exchange of bodily fluids during the delivery so the provider wants to know if there is a risk to the healthcare staff.
    c. The woman with HIV will be even more immunosuppressed during pregnancy so her status needs to be known.
    d. The woman with HIV disease can take antiretroviral agents during pregnancy to prevent maternal to fetal transmission in pregnancy.

65. A 30-year-old newly pregnant woman has a rapid plasma reagin test at the time of her first prenatal visit. Why is this test done?
    a. This will determine if she will pass on syphilis to her newborn at the time of delivery.
    b. This offers an opportunity to treat syphilis before it can be passed to the fetus in utero.
    c. This will identify those women who might have a preterm birth later in pregnancy.
    d. This will identify women who might develop tertiary syphilis during pregnancy.

66. The doctor is evaluating a woman who is in her first trimester and believes she has bacterial vaginosis. What is the most common symptom of the infection that would alert the woman she has the infection?
    a. Dysuria
    b. Perineal burning
    c. Low pelvic pain
    d. Malodorous vaginal discharge

67. A mother who is about to give birth asks you about neonatal infections. In discussing this, you tell her the most common serious infection in any newborn will likely be what?
    a. Listeriosis
    b. Group B streptococcus sepsis
    c. Gonorrhea sepsis
    d. Neurosyphilis

68. You are counseling a young woman who is in her first trimester as to how to avoid contraction Listeriosis. What is the main thing you say to her about avoiding the infection?
    a. Stay away from cow's milk
    b. Eat only cooked vegetables
    c. Stay away from processed luncheon meats
    d. Avoid eating at restaurants

69. You do not want a woman to have untreated syphilis while pregnant. What screening test is most used to check for this infection?
    a. Rapid plasma reagin test
    b. Anti-treponemal antibody test
    c. T pallidum test
    d. Chancre culture for treponemal organisms

70. You are caring for a 25-year-old woman who was found to have a positive culture for chlamydia in the middle of the third trimester. What is a first line agent for the treatment of this condition in pregnancy?
    a. Azithromycin
    b. Amoxicillin
    c. Erythromycin
    d. Ciprofloxacin

71. For what reason should a pregnant woman with a positive gonorrhea culture be given both a cephalosporin and azithromycin?
    a. Because there are a lot of drug resistances in gonorrheal infections.
    b. Because the two antibiotics act synergistically with one another.
    c. Because this enhances compliance with treatment.
    d. Because there is a high likelihood of a concomitant chlamydia infection that needs to be treated as well with azithromycin.

72. Women in pregnancy have an increased risk of urinary tract problems. What percentage of pregnant women will have asymptomatic bacteriuria at some point in their pregnancy?
    a. Five percent
    b. Ten percent
    c. Fifteen percent
    d. Twenty-five percent

73. You care for pregnant women, some of whom have genital infections. What is the most common presentation among pregnant women who have documented Chlamydia?
    a. Dysuria
    b. Cervical bleeding
    c. Yellow vaginal discharge
    d. No symptoms

74. You are caring for a recently pregnant mother who has just given birth and her infant quickly develops meningitis and grows Listeria out of the cerebrospinal fluid. What is the treatment of choice for this neonate?
    a. Intravenous ampicillin
    b. Oral trimethoprim/sulfamethoxazole
    c. Intravenous ciprofloxacin
    d. Intravenous vancomycin

75. Which historical statement is considered a risk factor for having a fraternal twin pregnancy?
    a. Having a history of infertility
    b. Having a history of pelvic inflammatory disease
    c. Being an older mother at the time of the pregnancy
    d. Having several previous childbirths

76. Why is it that many women in the first trimester of pregnancy with twins have greater symptoms of nausea and vomiting?
    a. The uterus is bigger and presses on the stomach.
    b. The levels of HCG are higher in twin gestations.
    c. The estradiol level is higher in twin gestations.
    d. The woman is less able to eat healthy foods when she is carrying twins.

77. At what time during a twin pregnancy will the pregnant woman feel the most active and will have the most energy?
    a. Sixth week gestation
    b. Tenth week gestation
    c. Fifteenth week gestation
    d. Twenty-seventh week gestation

78. When can the ultrasound technician use ultrasonography in a twin pregnancy to tell the mother what the genders are of her fetuses?
    a. Twelve to fourteen weeks
    b. Fourteen to sixteen weeks
    c. Sixteen to eighteen weeks
    d. Eighteen to twenty weeks

79. What is the most important thing for the obstetrician to follow in the third trimester in a twin gestation?
    a. Maternal weight gain
    b. Cervical dilatation status
    c. Maternal peripheral edema
    d. Maternal blood sugars

80. For what reason is that newly born twins remain in the hospital longer after birth when compared to singleton babies?
    a. They have a greater chance of neonatal infections
    b. They have more feeding difficulties
    c. They are smaller than singleton babies
    d. They have more complications related to being preterm

81. Which complication of pregnancy is more likely to occur in last several months of a twin pregnancy when compared to a singleton pregnancy?
    a. Group B strep colonization
    b. Gestational hypertension
    c. Chorioamnionitis
    d. Placental insufficiency

82. Why is it possible for a woman carrying twins to have problems walking in the third trimester of pregnancy?
    a. The uterus impairs the woman's full ability to take a deep breath
    b. The uterus is so heavy that the woman is clumsier than if she were carrying one baby
    c. There is a greater chance of separation of the pubic symphysis in a twin pregnancy
    d. The woman will have more peripheral edema with a twin pregnancy

83. What is the biggest complication in an identical twin pregnancy if there is documented twin-twin transfusion syndrome?

a. Both babies have a higher chance of being anemic.
   b. One baby will get too much blood while the other baby will get too little blood.
   c. One baby will be bigger than the other.
   d. One baby will survive while the other baby will die.

84. Why is a fraternal twin gestation considered safer for the babies than being a twin in an identical twin gestation?
    a. The fraternal twins will be less likely to be born preterm.
    b. The fraternal twins will have fewer respiratory complications than identical twins.
    c. Fraternal twins don't have problems related to twin-twin transfusion syndrome.
    d. Fraternal twins tend to be much larger at birth than identical twins.

85. What is usually the first sign that a woman is having a threatened spontaneous abortion?
    a. Low grade fever
    b. Vaginal bleeding
    c. Open cervix
    d. Lack of fetal heartbeat

86. Which is the most common presentation that can be found in a woman who has had a missed abortion?
    a. Vaginal bleeding
    b. Fever
    c. Coagulopathy of undetermined origin
    d. Diminishing signs of pregnancy

87. The woman you are managing has a mild placental abruption at 32-weeks' gestation. She is Rh negative. The placental abruption clots spontaneously and the pregnancy is allowed to continue. Without any medical intervention, what is the most serious complication of this pregnancy?
    a. Fetal demise from Rh sensitivity in the mother
    b. Small for gestational age infant
    c. Fetal developmental delay
    d. Chorioamnionitis later in pregnancy

88. The patient you are managing is a 22-year-old woman who has ultrasound evidence of an incomplete spontaneous abortion at 9 weeks' gestation. She wants to have the process over with and doesn't want to wait to see what happens. What medical therapy can you give her?
    a. Dilatation and curettage
    b. Misoprostol intravaginally
    c. Oxytocin intravenously
    d. Laminaria insertion

89. You are managing the healthcare of a woman who is being seen in the clinic for a three-week follow up visit after having a spontaneous abortion at 9 weeks' gestation, complicated by the need for a dilatation and curettage. What aspect of her care needs to be addressed the most?
    a. The provision of Rhogam
    b. Birth control option discussion
    c. Grief and loss issues
    d. Endometritis evaluation

90. The ultrasound has determined that a fetus has suffered a fetal demise at 41 weeks' gestation. Statistically, what is the most common cause of fetal demise at this gestational age?
    a. Chromosomal abnormalities
    b. Maternal smoking history
    c. Placental insufficiency
    d. Chorioamnionitis

91. The doctor is evaluating the status of a woman who has just had a completed miscarriage in her 10th week of gestation. This is the third time in a row that this has happened in the first trimester to this woman. What workup item should the doctor want to evaluate her for?
    a. Luteal phase defect
    b. Fetal karyotype for inherited chromosome abnormalities
    c. Cervical swab for HPV infection
    d. Incompetent cervix

92. The doctor is evaluating a 28-weeks' gestation pregnancy with an average-sized, active infant. The pregnancy is found to be complicated by oligohydramnios. The mother later presents to the hospital because of a lack of fetal movement. The fetus has no heartbeat on ultrasound. Statistically, what is the probable cause of this fetal demise?
    a. Fetal birth defect involving the kidneys
    b. Lack of fetal lung maturity
    c. Rh sensitization with fetal hydrops
    d. Umbilical cord accident

93. The doctor is giving advice to a nursing mother who has a three-month old infant. What type of birth control method can you recommend for her that will be the most effective in preventing a pregnancy?
    a. Fertility-based contraceptive techniques
    b. Breastfeeding to reduce fertility
    c. Progestin-only birth control pill
    d. Combination birth control pill

94. The doctor is caring for a 20-year-old woman who says she had unprotected intercourse five days ago and wants something to prevent a pregnancy. What can the doctor recommend for her?
    a. Plan B
    b. Single dose of ethynyl estradiol and norgestrel
    c. Combination birth control pills taken for the next five days at once per day
    d. Insertion of a copper T IUD

95. Why would a doctor caring for a young woman recommend that a 17-year-old girl using Norplant as a form of birth control also use condoms during sexual intercourse?
    a. The Norplant device has a modestly high failure rate so condoms can improve its effectiveness.
    b. Norplant doesn't protect against STDs so this high-risk woman should also use condoms.
    c. Norplant takes a couple of months to become effective so condoms are recommended.
    d. Norplant wears off after three months so it's a good idea to get into the habit of using condoms in case the follow up visits don't happen on schedule.

96. The doctor is caring for a woman with a history of a deep vein thrombosis in her leg five years ago who wishes birth control that will be effective and easy to remember. What birth control method might be suggested for her?
    a. Copper T IUD
    b. Ethynyl estradiol/norgestrel pills
    c. Diaphragm
    d. Cervical cap

97. The doctor is caring for a 14-year-old teen who wants something for birth control. She desires the Depo-Provera shot to be given every three months. What major side effect should be explained to her before giving her the shot?
    a. Heavy vaginal bleeding
    b. Weight gain
    c. Insulin resistance
    d. Vaginal dryness

98. What type of preoperative testing is imperative to do for a woman who is scheduled to have a tubal ligation within the next twenty-four hours?
    a. Ultrasound of the pelvis
    b. Serum progesterone level
    c. Serum HCG level
    d. Serum LH level

99. What kinds of medical risks does a woman face if she chooses to have a reversal of her tubal ligation?
    a. Primary ovarian failure
    b. Pelvic inflammatory disease
    c. Polycystic ovarian disease
    d. Ectopic pregnancy

100. Which birth control method listed below has the lowest typical use failure rate?
    a. Copper T IUD
    b. Mini-pill
    c. Depo-Provera injection
    d. Spermicidal jelly

Course Test Answers

1. When looking at a model of the female reproductive anatomy, where would you expect to find the bulk of the pubic hair?
    a. Mons pubis
    b. Labia minora
    c. Clitoris
    d. Labia majora

Answer: a. The mons pubis is just above the pubic symphysis and contains most of the woman's pubic hair.

2. When evaluating the female vagina, you notice structures that are believed to be stretch to allow for the passage of the fetus in the second stage of labor. What are these called?
    a. Suspensory ligaments
    b. Rugae
    c. Hymen
    d. Erectile tissues

Answer: b. When looking at the vagina, one can find rugae, which are folds of tissue that are highly distensible so they allow the vagina to dilate widely during the labor and delivery process.

3. Where during an evaluation of a woman's external genitalia would you most likely find an erectile structure?
    a. Hymen
    b. Labia minora
    c. Clitoris
    d. Skene gland

Answer: c. The clitoris is the primary erectile structure in the female reproductive organs.

4. Which structure in female reproductive anatomy can be found intact only when a young woman has not had the onset of menses?
    a. Clitoris
    b. Hymen
    c. Labia minora
    d. External os of the cervix

Answer: b. The hymen is a membranous covering that covers the vaginal opening in childhood. It needs to break to some degree to allow passage of menstrual blood and breaks completely at the time of first intercourse.

5. Which component of the female reproductive anatomy will change continuously throughout the month depending on the woman's hormone levels?
    a. Fallopian tubes
    b. Endometrium
    c. External cervical os

d. Vaginal rugae

Answer: b. The characteristics of the endometrium will change continuously and varies according to the hormonal changes associated with the menstrual cycle.

6. Approximately how many mature eggs does a woman's ovaries release as part of all the menstrual cycles she has during her lifetime?
    a. Fifty
    b. One hundred
    c. Three hundred
    d. One thousand

Answer: c. While there are millions of eggs in the female ovaries, only about three hundred mature eggs are released during all the ovulations a woman has in her lifetime.

7. The ovaries are suspended in several ways. Which ligament can be referred to as the suspensory ligament of the ovaries?
    a. Broad ligament
    b. Ovarian ligament
    c. Mesovarium
    d. Infundibular pelvic ligament

Answer: d. The infundibular pelvic ligament is responsible for suspending the ovaries in the pelvis. There is one such ligament for each of the woman's two ovaries.

8. When the ovaries are evaluated under the microscope, what histological finding is most likely to be identified?
    a. Sheets of immature egg cells in columns
    b. Connective tissue bands supporting immature egg cell structures
    c. Cystic structures of varying sizes representing follicles of different ages
    d. Scar tissue islands representing sclerosed follicles

Answer: c. Microscopic evaluation of the ovaries will show multiple cystic structures of varying sizes, which represent follicles of different ages.

9. You are doing a gross inspection of several female uteruses. Which patient would likely have the smallest uterine weight in grams?
    a. A pre-adolescent female
    b. A nulligravida 25-year-old female
    c. A multigravida 30-year-old female
    d. A 70-year-old postmenopausal female

Answer: d. Women who are no longer in their childbearing years will have a highly-atrophied uterus that will weigh much less than the uteruses of the younger women.

10. The doctor suspects that the woman is pregnant and performs an abdominal exam. She can palpate the uterus as being below the pubic symphysis. What can be inferred based on this examination?
    a. The woman has an ectopic pregnancy.

- b. The woman is in her second trimester of pregnancy.
- c. The woman is less than twelve weeks' gestation.
- d. The woman probably has an inevitable spontaneous abortion.

Answer: c. When the uterine fundus does not rise past the pubic symphysis, this is an indication that the pregnancy is less than twelve weeks' gestation. Bear in mind, however, that there is always the possibility of an ectopic pregnancy or spontaneous abortion that can't be ruled out based on this examination.

11. When examining a woman who is believed to be pregnant, the doctor notices a positive Chadwick sign. What causes this sign in pregnancy?
    - a. Venous congestion of the cervix
    - b. Thinning of the cervix
    - c. The presence of endometrial cells at the external os of the cervix
    - d. The presence of a cervix much lower in the vaginal canal than is seen in non-pregnant females

Answer: a. A positive Chadwick sign can be seen using a speculum exam and involves a bluish coloration of the cervix from increased venous congestion in pregnancy.

12. The doctor is examining the cervix while doing a bimanual examination on a 29-year-old female and detects a positive Hegar sign. At what gestational age should this sign be noticeable for the first time?
    - a. Four weeks' gestation
    - b. Six weeks' gestation
    - c. Eight weeks' gestation
    - d. Twelve weeks' gestation

Answer: b. A positive Hegar sign represents a softening of the cervix to palpation. It can easily be found on exam, beginning at about six weeks' gestation.

13. A newly pregnant woman has a serum HCG level of three hundred mIU per milliliter. In trying to decide if this is a false positive pregnancy test, what lab work can be done that will support the idea that the serum HCG level is a false positive test?
    - a. A serum progesterone level
    - b. A serum early pregnancy factor level
    - c. A urine qualitative pregnancy test
    - d. A repeat serum HCG level in two days

Answer: c. If it is believed that the serum HCG level is from a non-pregnancy source, repeating the test won't help show this and answers cannot be found in a serum progesterone level or in a serum early pregnancy factor level. On the other hand, a urine test for human chorionic gonadotropin is almost exclusively found in pregnancy so, if this is done, it can tell the difference between a pregnancy-related HCG elevation and a non-pregnancy-related HCG level.

14. The ultrasound technician is attempting to evaluate the viability of a fetus with a transvaginal ultrasound searching for a fetal heartbeat. At what fetal pole size should the heartbeat first be detected?

a. Two millimeters
b. Five millimeters
c. 50 millimeters
d. One centimeter

Answer: b. The heartbeat in the fetal pole can be first identified when the fetal pole is about five millimeters in diameter.

15. The doctor is trying to establish that a pregnancy is viable early in the first trimester. At what progesterone level can she be relatively assured of the existence of a healthy pregnancy?
    a. Five nanograms per milliliter
    b. Twenty-five nanograms per milliliter
    c. Fifty nanograms per milliliter
    d. Seventy-five nanograms per milliliter

Answer: d. The finding of a serum progesterone level of at least seventy-five nanograms per milliliter is usually a sign of a healthy intrauterine pregnancy, even early in the first trimester.

16. The technician is performing a transvaginal ultrasound on a woman believed to be newly pregnant. At what gestational age would the technician be able to see a fetal pole?
    a. Four to five weeks
    b. Five to six weeks
    c. Six to seven weeks
    d. Seven to eight weeks

Answer: b. A fetal pole can be identified first using a transvaginal ultrasound at about five to six weeks' gestational age.

17. Why is it a good idea to combine the technology of a transvaginal ultrasound along with HCG testing to identify a healthy pregnancy?
    a. Transvaginal ultrasounds are not very precise in identifying pregnancies before six weeks' gestation.
    b. The HCG level is better able to predict a healthy pregnancy when the ultrasound findings support the lab test.
    c. There are discriminatory levels that mean certain structures need to be present in a healthy pregnancy at certain HCG levels.
    d. The HCG alone cannot predict a healthy pregnancy.

Answer: c. Ultrasound and HCG testing can be helpful because there are certain discriminatory levels indicating when certain fetal structures can be seen at specific HCG levels.

18. Home pregnancy tests use a specific type of technology to detect a pregnancy. What type of technology do these tests utilize?
    a. Immunometric assay
    b. Immunoradiometric assay
    c. Enzyme-linked immunosorbent assay
    d. Radiometric assay

Answer: a. The urine home pregnancy test makes use of the immunometric assay. This type of testing isn't very sensitive, but it does not have the problem of false positive HCG levels that can be seen in serum testing.

19. The doctor is evaluating a woman regarding the cardiac changes seen in her pregnancy. Which statement about the heart changes in pregnancy is true?
    a. The stroke volume decreases
    b. The cardiac output increases
    c. The heart rate decreases
    d. The chances of arrhythmia are remote

Answer: b. During pregnancy, the cardiac output, stroke volume, and heart rate all go up in response to an increased need by the woman's circulation. At the same time, there is an increased chance of a benign arrhythmia.

20. The doctor performs a complete physical examination on a woman and finds that she has an enlarged thyroid gland and an elevated total thyroxine level in the second trimester of her pregnancy. What is the next thing that should be done to evaluate this finding?
    a. Perform a thyroid gland biopsy
    b. Obtain a radionuclide thyroid scan
    c. Obtain a total triiodothyronine level
    d. Do nothing as this is a physiological response in pregnancy

Answer: d. The finding of an enlarged thyroid gland and an elevated total thyroxine level in the second trimester of pregnancy is normal and is caused by the secretion of a TSH-like hormone by the placenta.

21. What is the specific action of progesterone on the maternal respiratory status?
    a. It decreases the partial pressure of oxygen
    b. It decreases the oxygen saturation
    c. It decreases the respiratory rate
    d. It decreases the carbon dioxide level

Answer: d. Progesterone will have the effect on the respiratory status by decreasing the carbon dioxide level in the bloodstream. This results in compensatory changes in the woman's respiratory system that act to keep a normal blood pH level.

22. What factors in the activities of a pregnant woman can cause an increase in kidney function?
    a. Lying on the left side
    b. Standing up
    c. Aerobically exercising
    d. Lying supine

Answer: b. When the pregnant woman lies on her left side, it causes increases the kidney function because it maximizes the circulation to the kidneys and increases the amount of water filtered through the kidneys.

23. What phenomenon explains the skin pigment changes seen in pregnancy?
    a. Increased risk of darkening of the skin from the sun

b. Increased keratinization of the skin tissues
   c. Increased melanocyte stimulating hormone
   d. Increased progesterone level from the placenta

Answer: c. The main thing that explains the pigment changes in the skin in pregnant women is the release of melanocyte stimulating hormone by the placenta. This acts on the melanocytes, which put out more of the melanin pigment.

24. If a serum prolactin level is drawn from the blood of a woman at thirty-six weeks' gestation, what would be expected regarding the result?
    a. A normal serum prolactin level as the patient hasn't breastfed yet
    b. A two-fold increase in the prolactin level
    c. A ten-fold increase in the prolactin level
    d. A one hundred-fold increase in the prolactin level

Answer: c. In pregnant women at term, a prolactin level, if one would be drawn, would show a ten-fold increase in serum prolactin that quickly normalizes shortly after childbirth, even in women who are lactating.

25. Why is there frequently the finding of peripheral edema in an examination of a pregnant woman?
    a. A decrease in the glomerular filtration rate
    b. An increase in water and salt uptake by the kidneys
    c. A decrease in serum aldosterone levels
    d. An increase in serum progesterone levels

Answer: b. Pregnant women can get peripheral edema because they have an increase in water and salt uptake by the kidneys. The kidneys are influenced by increased aldosterone and cortisol levels in pregnancy, which are elevated by the placental production of corticotropin releasing hormone.

26. What gross physical finding may be present in a woman's urinary tract system while she is pregnant?
    a. An enlargement of both kidneys
    b. A shrinkage of the bladder
    c. An enlargement of the ureters
    d. A foreshortening of the urethra

Answer: c. The most obvious gross physical finding seen in the urinary tract of pregnant women is hydroureter or massive enlargement of the ureters.

27. What is the primary cause of breast engorgement and tenderness among women who are in the early stages of pregnancy?
    a. Elevated progesterone levels
    b. Elevated HCG levels
    c. Elevated estradiol levels
    d. Elevated prolactin levels

Answer: c. Elevated estradiol levels, which rise dramatically after the woman misses her period, will result in breast engorgement and tenderness that tends to go away sometime in the first trimester of pregnancy.

28. Why is insulin resistance a natural part of the physiology of a pregnant woman?
    a. Increased estradiol levels
    b. Increased cortisol levels
    c. Increased HCG levels
    d. Increased alkaline phosphatase levels

Answer: b. Pregnant women have increased cortisol levels, which result in insulin resistance. This can lead to gestational diabetes or worsening of diabetes in women who had insulin resistance prior to the pregnancy.

29. When is it a good idea for a woman to schedule a pre-pregnancy gynecological visit?
    a. Only if she is older than thirty-five years of age
    b. Only if she suffers from infertility
    c. Only if she has an underlying medical problem before becoming pregnant
    d. Any time a woman wants to make sure she is healthy enough for a pregnancy

Answer: d. The pre-pregnancy gynecological visit is not mandatory, but it should be scheduled anytime the woman wants to ensure she is healthy enough to become pregnant.

30. When in a woman's pregnancy is the maternal screening test for gestational diabetes performed?
    a. At the first prenatal visit
    b. Anytime sugar is found in the urine
    c. At twenty-four weeks
    d. At thirty-two weeks

Answer: c. The gestational diabetes screening test is done on all pregnant women at twenty-four weeks' gestation. Some women are tested before that time if there is evidence to suggest the woman has gestational diabetes.

31. Preterm labor can be defined as any labor that occurs before which gestational age?
    a. Twenty-eight weeks
    b. Thirty-two weeks
    c. Thirty-five weeks
    d. Thirty-seven weeks

Answer: d. Preterm labor is defined as any labor resulting in cervical changes before the thirty-seventh week of pregnancy.

32. What laboratory study is not tested as part of the triple screen?
    a. Fetal karyotype
    b. Human chorionic gonadotropin
    c. Alpha fetoprotein
    d. Conjugated estriol

Answer: a. All the above choices are performed as part of the triple screen except for the fetal karyotype, which is not a blood test at all.

33. When in a woman's pregnancy does an amniocentesis usually occur if this test is found to be necessary?
    a. Ten to twelve weeks
    b. Fourteen to sixteen weeks
    c. Eighteen to twenty weeks
    d. Twenty to twenty-two weeks

Answer: c. When indicated, the amniocentesis is generally performed between eighteen and twenty weeks' gestation.

34. Pregnant women often get heartburn. Which recommendation could be given to help reduce this symptom?
    a. Take an antacid with every meal
    b. Avoid taking aspirin
    c. Elevate the head of the bed at night
    d. Eat a high protein diet

Answer: c. Something that can be done to reduce heartburn is to elevate the head of the bed at night, which keeps the stomach contents from rising into the esophagus.

35. A woman asks what she can do to avoid getting the Zika virus. What can she do to reduce her risk?
    a. Avoid unwashed vegetables
    b. Avoid processed lunchmeats
    c. Avoid travel to endemic countries
    d. Avoid intercourse with anyone other than her sexual partner

Answer: c. Pregnant patients who want to avoid the Zika virus can do this simply by avoiding unnecessary travel to countries in which the virus is prevalent. It is passed through a mosquito bite but rarely can be passed through sexual intercourse.

36. What is the best description of the four-dimensional ultrasound?
    a. It gives snapshots of the fetus's structures using sound waves
    b. It gives intricate detail of the fetus's inner organs
    c. It gives realistic pictures of the fetus's facial features
    d. It combines images of the fetus and evaluates fetal movements

Answer: d. The four-dimensional ultrasound provides clear images of the fetus and evaluates fetal movements at the same time.

37. A woman being seen in labor is six centimeters dilated and is experiencing a slowdown in the strength and frequency of her contractions. What first step can you do that will increase the rate of her contractions?
    a. Have her sit on the toilet
    b. Perform an amniotomy
    c. Add IV fluids to her treatment plan

d. Give prostaglandin E2 gel to the cervix

Answer: b. An amniotomy can easily be performed and will break the bag of water. Doing this alone will generally stimulate contractions, particularly if the woman is in the active phase of the first stage of labor.

38. Why shouldn't the obstetrician or family doctor do an amniotomy in the latent phase of labor in an HIV-infected mother?
    a. It will increase her bleeding risk.
    b. It increases the chance of getting chorioamnionitis.
    c. It tends not to increase the strength and frequency of her contractions.
    d. It increases the fetus's exposure to the HIV virus in utero.

Answer: d. An amniotomy or rupture of membranes should be done as late as possible or not at all in HIV-infected mothers. This is because doing so causes a longer exposure time for the fetus to be in contact with the maternal blood, when they can contract HIV as a neonate.

39. The woman is being seen in the labor and delivery unit and is in the first stage of labor. What clinical finding warrants further investigation?
    a. A sudden gush of clear fluid from the vagina
    b. A maternal temperature of 99.0 degrees Fahrenheit
    c. Continuous abdominal pain
    d. Increased urinary frequency

Answer: c. Continuous abdominal pain is not normal in the first stage of labor and might mean chorioamnionitis or an abrupted placenta. This finding requires further intervention.

40. The doctor believes that a woman in the second stage of labor needs an episiotomy. What is the main advantage of doing a mediolateral episiotomy?
    a. It is technically easier to do
    b. The blood loss is less
    c. There is less pain with this type of episiotomy
    d. There is no chance of extension into the rectum

Answer: a. The major advantage of doing a mediolateral episiotomy is that it is technically easier to perform. The blood loss can be more with this type and the pain is often greater. It still has the potential to extend into the rectum but to a lesser degree than is true of a midline episiotomy.

41. The doctor is examining a pregnant woman at term before she goes into labor and suspects there will be shoulder dystocia. What things might lead the doctor to be prepared for this obstetrical complication?
    a. Previous baby weighing nine pounds
    b. Gestational diabetes
    c. Onset of labor at thirty-seven weeks
    d. Male gender of the fetus

Answer: b. Women with gestational diabetes often have very large babies and put themselves at risk of having shoulder dystocia after the successful delivery of the fetal head.

42. Why might the doctor choose to tell the laboring woman to wait on pushing in the second stage until there is bulging of the perineum?
   a. Pushing too early can lead to fetal distress
   b. Pushing late in the second stage provides less blood loss
   c. Pushing late in the second stage provides for more effective pushing
   d. The baby will be delivered just as quickly if she waits

Answer: c. Some doctors prefer the woman wait to push until the perineum is bulging, which gives a stronger urge to push and facilitate more effective pushing.

43. What is the most common cause of bleeding in the third stage of labor?
   a. Retained placenta or placental fragments
   b. Uterine laceration
   c. Cervical laceration
   d. Full bladder

Answer: a. The most common cause of bleeding in the third stage of labor is a retained placenta or retained placental fragments, although any of the other choices might also cause bleeding to occur.

44. The doctor is managing a woman who has sustained a postpartum hemorrhage. What is the definition of a postpartum hemorrhage?
   a. She has lost blood after the delivery of the placenta
   b. She required blood transfusions after the delivery
   c. She lost more than 500 milliliters of blood in twenty-four hours
   d. She required intraoperative intervention to control bleeding

Answer: c. The basic definition of a postpartum hemorrhage is having lost 500 milliliters of blood within the first twenty-four hours after childbirth. It can be from many causes.

45. During the examination of the placenta after birth, a firm blood clot on the side of the placenta that had been attached to the uterine wall is visualized. What can this mean?
   a. The patient has a cotyledon left in the placenta
   b. The woman has normal clotting factors and doesn't have a bleeding disorder
   c. She had an area of placental infarction near term
   d. She had a partially abrupted placenta near term

Answer: d. The patient with a blood clot adherent to the placenta likely had a partial abruption at the time of labor or shortly before going into labor.

46. A new mother is being evaluated prior to being discharged from the hospital after an uncomplicated vaginal delivery. If the mother and infant are stable, what is the accepted minimum amount of time the woman should be in the hospital before allowing her to go home?
   a. Three hours
   b. Six hours
   c. Twelve hours
   d. Forty-eight hours

Answer: b. Women should stay in the hospital or birthing center for at least six hours after giving birth, but can be discharged thereafter if they are medically stable.

47. A woman presents to the emergency room with the sudden onset of a red, tender breast and a fever. She is breastfeeding a two-week-old infant. How should this woman's problem be addressed?
    a. Restrict breastfeeding to the normal breast until the infection resolves.
    b. Instruct the woman to use hot compresses on the affected breast.
    c. Provide the woman with an antibiotic that does not penetrate breast milk.
    d. Provide the woman with an antibiotic that is safe when ingested by the newborn.

Answer: d. The woman who is nursing a baby and who has mastitis should be allowed to continue breastfeeding on the affected breast and should be given an antibiotic that is safely ingested by newborns.

48. A 30-year old woman is being seen in the clinic. She is nursing her two-month-old infant and wants something for birth control. What is the most effective birth control method you can prescribe or recommend for her?
    a. Diaphragm
    b. Male condom
    c. Mini-pill
    d. Estradiol/Progestin pill

Answer: c. The safest and most effective form of birth control for a nursing mother is the mini-pill, which contains only progestins and can be ingested by the breastfeeding infant.

49. The patient is a 35-year-old woman who is breastfeeding and has clinical signs and symptoms of postpartum depression. What treatment can be given safely to her while she breastfeeds?
    a. Nortriptyline
    b. Amitriptyline
    c. Fluoxetine
    d. Electroconvulsive therapy

Answer: d. A breastfeeding mother can have antidepressants while nursing but there is always going to be a risk to the infant by doing so. For this reason, the safest option is to use electroconvulsive therapy, which does not harm the infant in any way.

50. The patient in question has just had a vaginal delivery. At what time can you expect her uterus to shrink to its pre-pregnancy size?
    a. Two weeks
    b. Four weeks
    c. Six weeks
    d. It will never shrink to the pre-pregnancy size

Answer: d. While the uterus will continue to shrink until six weeks' postpartum, it will never actually shrink to its pre-pregnancy size after a woman has given birth.

51. A woman being seen by a visiting home nurse is one week postpartum and has symptoms of tearfulness and low mood that have not impacted her sleep, appetite, or her care of her newborn. The nurse can tell the woman these symptoms are likely to last for how long?
    a. Two weeks
    b. Six weeks
    c. Two months
    d. Six months

Answer: a. The woman is exhibiting classical symptoms of the baby blues. These symptoms generally only last for two weeks after the birth of the child and spontaneously improve without treatment.

52. The husband of a postpartum woman calls to say his wife is hallucinating and has illogical thoughts. She is unable to care for her infant and he needs to do all the childcare. What advice should you give him?
    a. He should make an appointment for his wife to see a psychiatrist.
    b. He should start giving her an antipsychotic drug that you will provide for her.
    c. He needs to have her seen urgently in the emergency department.
    d. He needs to pick up a prescription for an antidepressant medication to give her.

Answer: c. The woman with these symptoms likely has postpartum psychosis, which is a psychiatric emergency requiring urgent medical attention. She needs to be seen in the emergency department and probably admitted to a locked psychiatric unit.

53. When talking about postpartum depression with a woman who is having the symptoms of the disorder, what do you tell her the incidence is of this problem among postpartum women?
    a. One to two percent
    b. Four to six percent
    c. Ten to twenty percent
    d. Twenty to thirty percent

Answer: c. The incidence of postpartum depression among women who have just given birth is about ten to twenty percent. For this reason, this disorder must be screened for in every woman who has recently given birth.

54. The doctor's job is to discuss birth control methods and contraception with all postpartum patients. At what point after childbirth should this discussion take place?
    a. At the time of hospital discharge
    b. At two weeks' postpartum
    c. At the six-week postpartum visit
    d. By the sixth postpartum month

Answer: a. As a woman can get pregnant before her six-week postpartum visit, a discussion regarding birth control options should take place prior to her discharge from the hospital. Any time after that may be too late to initiate adequate contraception.

55. A postpartum mother presents to the clinic with the complaint of constipation after having an unremarkable vaginal delivery without an episiotomy the week before. What can be recommended for her that will help this problem?
    a. Bisacodyl suppositories
    b. Fluids and increased fiber
    c. Milk of Magnesia
    d. Mylanta

Answer: b. In most cases of constipation after childbirth, nothing is required after giving birth apart from increasing fluids and adding fiber to the diet.

56. A pregnant woman is in her third trimester and is found on examination to have a resting blood pressure of 165/100. What is the next test that should be done to evaluate this finding?
    a. Electrocardiogram
    b. Brachial ankle index
    c. Urine dipstick for protein
    d. Serum protein level

Answer: c. What isn't known is whether the patients hypertension is essential hypertension, gestational hypertension, or preeclampsia. The test that can help define this is a urine dipstick for protein, which will show protein in the urine in cases of preeclampsia.

57. The woman being evaluated in the emergency department is 32-weeks' gestational age with a blood pressure reading of 155/95. The urinalysis shows 3+ protein in the urine. What can be given to prevent eclampsia?
    a. IV nitroprusside
    b. Oral labetalol
    c. IV hydralazine
    d. IV magnesium sulfate

Answer: d. While any of the antihypertensive medications listed can easily bring the blood pressure down, they don't do anything to prevent the seizures associated with eclampsia. Only intravenous magnesium sulfate can do this.

58. The woman being seen in the hospital is a 32-year-old multiparous woman with preeclampsia. When can she be safely assured of having no neurological complication from this problem?
    a. As soon as her blood pressure reaches below the 140/90 threshold
    b. As soon as she delivers her infant
    c. About three to four days after delivery
    d. After receiving at least forty-eight hours of labetalol orally

Answer: c. The woman's chance of seizures will be present until about three to four days after the delivery.

59. The patient is a primiparous woman who is having routine prenatal care. As part of this care, when should she have a one-hour glucose tolerance test for gestational diabetes?
    a. First prenatal visit
    b. Twelve weeks' gestational age
    c. Eighteen weeks' gestational age
    d. Twenty-four weeks' gestational age

Answer: d. A pregnant woman should receive a one-hour glucose tolerance test for gestational diabetes at twenty-four weeks' gestational age unless there is evidence that she has the disorder earlier in the pregnancy by history or lab findings.

60. A woman with type 2 diabetes on metformin becomes pregnant and sees her primary care physician for management of her diabetes. How will her diabetes be managed during the pregnancy?
    a. She will remain on metformin but will monitor her blood sugars three times a day.
    b. She will stop the metformin and start a program of insulin therapy.
    c. She will stop the metformin and will begin a strict diet and exercise program for her diabetes.
    d. She will check blood sugars four times daily and will switch to Victoza (liraglutide)

Answer: b. Pregnant women with any type of diabetes need to be on insulin therapy for the duration of their pregnancy as the oral drugs for diabetes are not considered as safe to be used in pregnant women.

61. A 30-year-old overweight female is in her first trimester of pregnancy and has a baseline history of hypertension. In managing her hypertension in pregnancy, what would a first line medication be for this?
    a. Labetalol
    b. Nifedipine
    c. Captopril
    d. Losartan

Answer: a. Labetalol is considered a first line agent for the management of hypertension in pregnancy. Nifedipine can be used for postpartum hypertension. Captopril and Losartan are contraindicated in pregnancy and should not be used.

62. The doctor is caring for an infant who was born to a mother has known chronic hepatitis B. How is this handled?
    a. The infant is given the hepatitis B vaccine at two weeks of age.
    b. The infant is tested for the virus and, if negative, is given the hepatitis B vaccine.
    c. The infant is given the hepatitis B immune globulin.
    d. The infant is given the hepatitis B immune globulin and the hepatitis B vaccine on the day of birth.

Answer: d. If an infant is born to a mother known to have chronic hepatitis B, the infant should receive the hepatitis B immune globulin at the time of birth and should be vaccinated against hepatitis B within 12 hours of birth.

63. The doctor is caring for an infant who was born to a mother who had an active gonorrhea infection at the time of a vaginal birth. How should the infant be treated?
    a. The infant is given oral systemic antibiotics against gonorrhea.
    b. A blood culture is obtained, and the infant is treated if positive for gonorrhea.
    c. The infant is given erythromycin eye drops to protect against gonorrhea conjunctivitis.
    d. The infant is intravenous antibiotics against gonorrhea.

Answer: a. Whenever an infant is born to a mother known to have vaginal or cervical gonorrhea, the infant and the mother should receive oral systemic coverage for the gonorrhea infection.

64. The doctor is caring for a pregnant woman who tested positive for HIV at the time of her first prenatal visit. For what reason is this test done on all pregnant women?
    a. Many pregnant women are high risk for HIV, so they should be screened whenever they become pregnant.
    b. There will be a lot of exchange of bodily fluids during the delivery, so the provider wants to know if there is a risk to the healthcare staff.
    c. The woman with HIV will be even more immunosuppressed during pregnancy so her status needs to be known.
    d. The woman with HIV disease can take antiretroviral agents during pregnancy to prevent maternal to fetal transmission.

Answer: d. Any woman who has HIV disease in pregnancy can take antiretroviral agents during pregnancy to prevent maternal to fetal transmission.

65. A 30-year-old newly pregnant woman has a rapid plasma reagin test at the time of her first prenatal visit. Why is this test done?
    a. This will determine if she will pass on syphilis to her newborn at the time of delivery.
    b. This offers an opportunity to treat syphilis before it can be passed to the fetus in utero.
    c. This will identify women who might have a preterm birth later in pregnancy.
    d. This will identify women who might develop tertiary syphilis during pregnancy.

Answer: b. Testing for syphilis with a rapid plasma reagin test will allow a woman to be treated for syphilis before the disease can be passed to the fetus.

66. The doctor is evaluating a woman who is in her first trimester and believes she has bacterial vaginosis. What is the most common symptom of the infection that would alert the woman she has the infection?
    a. Dysuria
    b. Perineal burning
    c. Low pelvic pain
    d. Malodorous vaginal discharge

Answer: d. There aren't many symptoms associated with bacterial vaginosis. The main symptom noted by women is a malodorous vaginal discharge that often smells like fish.

67. A mother who is about to give birth asks you about neonatal infections. In discussing this, you tell her the most common serious infection in any newborn will likely be what?
    a. Listeriosis
    b. Group B streptococcus sepsis
    c. Gonorrhea sepsis
    d. Neurosyphilis

Answer: b. The most common serious infection in neonates is group B streptococcus sepsis. The other infections are much less likely to occur in neonates.

68. You are counseling a young woman who is in her first trimester as to how to avoid contracting Listeriosis. What is the main thing you say to her about avoiding the infection?
    a. Stay away from cow's milk
    b. Eat only cooked vegetables
    c. Stay away from processed lunch meats
    d. Avoid eating at restaurants

Answer: c. Because the Listeria infection can come from processed lunch meats that haven't been properly handled, pregnant women should avoid eating processed lunch meats.

69. You do not want a woman to have untreated syphilis while pregnant. What screening test is most commonly used to check for this infection?
    a. Rapid plasma reagin test
    b. Anti-treponemal antibody test
    c. T pallidum test
    d. Chancre culture for treponemal organisms

Answer: a. The primary screening test for syphilis is the rapid plasma reagin test. The other tests can be confirmatory or aren't used in the screening of patients for syphilis.

70. You are caring for a 25-year-old woman who was found to have a positive culture for chlamydia in the middle of the third trimester. What is a first line agent for the treatment of this condition in pregnancy?
    a. Azithromycin
    b. Amoxicillin
    c. Erythromycin
    d. Ciprofloxacin

Answer: a. Azithromycin is the first like agent for the treatment of chlamydia in pregnancy. The other choices are not first line agents or are contraindicated in pregnancy.

71. For what reason should a pregnant woman with a positive gonorrhea culture be given both a cephalosporin and azithromycin?
    a. Because there are a lot of drug resistances in gonorrheal infections.
    b. Because the two antibiotics act synergistically with one another.
    c. Because this enhances compliance with treatment.
    d. Because there is a high likelihood of a concomitant chlamydia infection that needs to be treated as well with azithromycin.

Answer: d. Women with a positive gonorrhea culture in pregnancy have a high risk of also having a chlamydia infection so empiric coverage for chlamydia is done even if it was not cultured or otherwise identified.

72. Women in pregnancy have an increased risk of urinary tract problems. What percentage of pregnant women will have asymptomatic bacteriuria at some point in their pregnancy?
    a. Five percent
    b. Ten percent
    c. Fifteen percent
    d. Twenty-five percent

Answer: c. Up to fifteen percent of pregnant women will have asymptomatic bacteriuria during pregnancy so cultures of the urine should be performed at least once as part of good prenatal care.

73. What is the most common presentation among pregnant women who have documented Chlamydia?
    a. Dysuria
    b. Cervical bleeding
    c. Yellow vaginal discharge
    d. No symptoms

Answer: d. Up to seventy-five percent of pregnant women with chlamydia will have no symptoms.

74. You are caring for a recently pregnant mother who has just given birth and her infant quickly develops meningitis and grows Listeria out of the cerebrospinal fluid. What is the treatment of choice for this neonate?
    a. Intravenous ampicillin
    b. Oral trimethoprim/sulfamethoxazole
    c. Intravenous ciprofloxacin
    d. Intravenous vancomycin

Answer: a. The treatment of choice for a pregnant mother or her infant who have documented listeria infections is to give intravenous ampicillin, particularly for neonatal meningitis.

75. Which historical statement is considered a risk factor for having a fraternal twin pregnancy?
    a. Having a history of infertility
    b. Having a history of pelvic inflammatory disease
    c. Being an older mother at the time of the pregnancy
    d. Having several previous childbirths

Answer: c. Being an older mother at the time of pregnancy is a risk factor for having fraternal twins as older women are more likely to release more than one egg at a time.

76. Why is it that many women in the first trimester of pregnancy with twins have greater symptoms of nausea and vomiting?
    a. The uterus is bigger and presses on the stomach.
    b. The levels of HCG are higher in twin gestations.
    c. The estradiol level is higher in twin gestations.

d. The woman is less able to eat healthy foods when she is carrying twins.

Answer: b. Twin pregnancies have higher HCG levels. HCG levels are directly associated with the level of nausea and vomiting so, in pregnancies with twins, the risk of these symptoms is greater.

77. At what time during a twin pregnancy will the pregnant woman feel the most active and will have the most energy?
    a. Sixth week gestation
    b. Tenth week gestation
    c. Fifteenth week gestation
    d. Twenty-seventh week gestation

Answer: c. Women in the second trimester of a twin pregnancy with often experiance much less fatigue and feel more energized, with an increase in activity level.

78. When can the ultrasound technician use ultrasonography in a twin pregnancy to tell the mother what the genders are of her fetuses?
    a. Twelve to fourteen weeks
    b. Fourteen to sixteen weeks
    c. Sixteen to eighteen weeks
    d. Eighteen to twenty weeks

Answer: d. The gender of the fetus can be accurately determined between the eighteenth to twentieth weeks' gestation.

79. What is the most important thing for the obstetrician to follow in the third trimester in a twin gestation?
    a. Maternal weight gain
    b. Cervical dilatation status
    c. Maternal peripheral edema
    d. Maternal blood sugars

Answer: b. The most important thing to evaluate is the cervical dilatation status as this is an indicator of the possibility of a preterm birth.

80. For what reason do newly born twins remain in the hospital longer after birth when compared to singleton babies?
    a. They have a greater chance of neonatal infections
    b. They have more feeding difficulties
    c. They are smaller than singleton babies
    d. They have more complications related to being preterm

Answer: d. Twins are more likely to be preterm at birth and will spend more time in the neonatal intensive care unit with complications related to being preterm. This means they will be in the hospital longer than most singleton babies.

81. Which complication of pregnancy is more likely to occur in the last several months of a twin pregnancy when compared to a singleton pregnancy?
    a. Group B strep colonization

b. Gestational hypertension
c. Chorioamnionitis
d. Placental insufficiency

Answer: b. Gestational hypertension is a complication of the last several months of pregnancy that tends to occur more likely in women carrying twins when compared to a singleton pregnancy.

82. Why does a woman carrying twins often have problems walking in the third trimester of pregnancy?
    a. The uterus impairs the woman's full ability to take a deep breath
    b. The uterus is so heavy that the woman is clumsier than if she were carrying one baby
    c. There is a greater chance of separation of the pubic symphysis in a twin pregnancy
    d. The woman will have more peripheral edema with a twin pregnancy

Answer: c. The heavier uterus in a twin pregnancy will put more pressure on the woman's pelvis, increasing her chances of having a separation of the pubic symphysis, which makes walking more difficult.

83. What is the biggest complication in an identical twin pregnancy if there is documented twin-twin transfusion syndrome?
    a. Both babies have a higher chance of being anemic.
    b. One baby will get too much blood while the other baby will get too little blood.
    c. One baby will be bigger than the other.
    d. One baby will survive while the other baby will die.

Answer: b. Twin-twin transfusion syndrome is a serious complication of identical twin pregnancies when one twin gets too much blood and one twin gets too little blood. It does not necessarily cause the death of either twin if managed appropriately.

84. Why is a fraternal twin gestation considered safer for the babies than being a twin in an identical twin gestation?
    a. The fraternal twins will be less likely to be born preterm.
    b. The fraternal twins will have fewer respiratory complications than identical twins.
    c. Fraternal twins don't have problems related to twin-twin transfusion syndrome.
    d. Fraternal twins tend to be much larger at birth than identical twins.

Answer: c. Fraternal twins have their own placenta, their own umbilical cord, and their own amniotic sac so there isn't the problem with twin-twin transfusion syndrome that can complicate an identical twin pregnancy.

85. What is usually the first sign that a woman is having a threatened spontaneous abortion?
    a. Low grade fever
    b. Vaginal bleeding
    c. Open cervix
    d. Lack of fetal heartbeat

Answer: b. Generally, the first finding in a threatened spontaneous abortion is vaginal bleeding.

86. Which is the most common presentation in a woman with a missed abortion?

a. Vaginal bleeding
b. Fever
c. Coagulopathy of undetermined origin
d. Diminishing signs of pregnancy

Answer: d. A missed abortion means that the embryo or fetus has died but remains in the uterus. There may be no bleeding and there is no cramping. The only symptom may be a lack of pregnancy symptoms that were present before the fetal loss.

87. The woman you are managing has a mild placental abruption at 32-weeks' gestation. She is Rh-negative. The placental abruption clots spontaneously and the pregnancy is allowed to continue. Without any medical intervention, what is the most serious complication of this pregnancy?
    a. Fetal demise from Rh sensitivity in the mother
    b. Small for gestational age infant
    c. Fetal developmental delay
    d. Chorioamnionitis later in pregnancy

Answer: a. The most serious complication of a placental abruption in an Rh-negative mother is the mixing of maternal and fetal blood, causing fetal demise from Rh sensitization in the mother.

88. The patient you are managing is a 22-year-old woman who has ultrasound evidence of an incomplete spontaneous abortion at 9 weeks' gestation. She does not want to wait for the products of conception to pass on their own. What medical therapy can you give her?
    a. Dilatation and curettage
    b. Misoprostol intravaginally
    c. Oxytocin intravenously
    d. Laminaria insertion

Answer: b. Misoprostol is a small pill that can be given intravaginally. It will help open the cervix and will stimulate contractions and cramping that will expel the products of conception. Oxytocin will be ineffective at this point and the other choices are not considered medical interventions.

89. You are seeing a woman in the clinic for her three-week follow up visit after having a spontaneous abortion at 9 weeks' gestation, complicated by the need for a dilatation and curettage. What aspect of her care should be addressed the most?
    a. The provision of Rhogam
    b. Birth control option discussion
    c. Grief and loss issues
    d. Endometritis evaluation

Answer: c. At three weeks after a dilatation and curettage for a miscarriage, the chances of endometritis are remote. Rhogam should have already been given at the time of the procedure. Birth control options are much less of a priority than issues around grief and loss.

90. The ultrasound has determined that a fetus has suffered a fetal demise at 41 weeks' gestation. Statistically, what is the most common cause of fetal demise at this gestational age?
    a. Chromosomal abnormalities
    b. Maternal smoking history

c. Placental insufficiency
d. Chorioamnionitis

Answer: c. At 41 to 42 weeks' gestation, the most common reason for a fetal demise is placental insufficiency because the placenta has gotten so old that it cannot provide adequate amounts of nutrients and oxygen to the fetus.

91. The doctor is evaluating the status of a woman who has just had a completed miscarriage in her 10th week of gestation. This is the third time in a row that this has happened in the first trimester to this woman. What should doctor evaluate this woman for?
    a. Luteal phase defect
    b. Fetal karyotype for inherited chromosome abnormalities
    c. Cervical swab for HPV infection
    d. Incompetent cervix

Answer: b. As all the woman's miscarriages are in the first trimester, they are not likely to be due to an incompetent cervix. A luteal phase defect will be problematic in extremely early pregnancy losses. HPV infections do not cause recurrent miscarriages but abnormalities in the fetal karyotype or parental karyotypes might point to a specific chromosomal abnormality causing the pregnancy losses.

92. The doctor is evaluating a 28-weeks' gestation pregnancy with an average-sized, active infant. The pregnancy is complicated by oligohydramnios. The mother later presents to the hospital because of a lack of fetal movement. The fetus has no heartbeat on ultrasound. Statistically, what is the most probable cause of this fetal demise?
    a. Fetal birth defect involving the kidneys
    b. Lack of fetal lung maturity
    c. Rh sensitization with fetal hydrops
    d. Umbilical cord accident

Answer: d. In a pregnancy near term with oligohydramnios, the cord has very little space in which to float freely. This increases the likelihood of a cord accident. The other choices are not complications of oligohydramnios that lead to fetal demise in utero.

93. The doctor is giving advice to a nursing mother who has a three-month old infant. What type of birth control method can you recommend that will be the most effective in preventing a pregnancy?
    a. Fertility-based contraceptive techniques
    b. Breastfeeding to reduce fertility
    c. Progestin-only birth control pill
    d. Combination birth control pill

Answer: c. Women who are breastfeeding and want a hormonal birth control option that will be very effective in preventing a pregnancy can take a progestin-only birth control pill, which is also called the mini-pill.

94. The doctor is caring for a 20-year-old woman who says she had unprotected intercourse five days ago and wants something to prevent a pregnancy. What can the doctor recommend for her?
    a. Plan B
    b. Single dose of ethynyl estradiol and norgestrel
    c. Combination birth control pills taken for the next five days at once per day
    d. Insertion of a copper T IUD

Answer: d. All hormonal methods of emergency contraception tend only to be effective if used within seventy-two hours after intercourse. The Copper T IUD can be used if placed within five days of unprotected intercourse and is the treatment of choice.

95. Why would a doctor caring for a young woman recommend that a 17-year-old girl using Norplant as a form of birth control also use condoms during sexual intercourse?
    a. The Norplant device has a modestly high failure rate, so condoms can improve its effectiveness.
    b. Norplant doesn't protect against STDs, so this high-risk woman should also use condoms.
    c. Norplant takes a couple of months to become effective, so condoms are recommended.
    d. Norplant wears off after three months so it's a good idea to get into the habit of using condoms in case the follow up visits don't happen on schedule.

Answer: b. Norplant is extremely effective alone in preventing pregnancy, but it does not protect against STDs. For this reason, condoms should be recommended in high-risk women and teens.

96. The doctor is caring for a woman with a history of a deep vein thrombosis in her leg five years ago who seeks birth control that will be effective and easy to remember. What birth control method might be suggested for her?
    a. Copper T IUD
    b. Ethynyl estradiol/norgestrel pills
    c. Diaphragm
    d. Cervical cap

Answer: a. This is a woman who is at a high risk of getting another DVT if she takes birth control pills and should be offered a birth control option that has a low failure rate. She can't take any estrogen-containing birth control pill; however, the copper T IUD is highly effective, easy to remember, and won't adversely affect her blood clotting risk.

97. The doctor is caring for a 14-year-old teen who wants something for birth control. She desires the Depo-Provera shot to be given every three months. What major side effect should be explained to her before giving her the shot?
    a. Heavy vaginal bleeding
    b. Weight gain
    c. Insulin resistance

d. Vaginal dryness

Answer: b. The major side effect of Depo-Provera is weight gain. Teens may decide not to follow through with tri-monthly injections if they find it is causing them to gain weight, so they need to be informed about this side effect in advance.

98. What type of preoperative testing is imperative to do for a woman who is scheduled to have a tubal ligation within the next twenty-four hours?
    a. Ultrasound of the pelvis
    b. Serum progesterone level
    c. Serum HCG level
    d. Serum LH level

Answer: c. A serum HCG level should be done to rule out a pregnancy before doing the tubal ligation. Ideally, the testing should be done after a menstrual period but before ovulation has taken place and the tubal ligation should be done in the first part of the menstrual cycle.

99. What kinds of medical risks does a woman face if she chooses to have a reversal of her tubal ligation?
    a. Primary ovarian failure
    b. Pelvic inflammatory disease
    c. Polycystic ovarian disease
    d. Ectopic pregnancy

Answer: d. Because it is not possible to have completely smooth fallopian tube walls after repair of a previous tubal ligation, the egg or embryo can get stuck in the fallopian tube, resulting in an ectopic pregnancy.

100. Which birth control method listed below has the lowest typical use failure rate?
    a. Copper T IUD
    b. Mini-pill
    c. Depo-Provera injection
    d. Spermicidal jelly

Answer: a. The Copper T IUD has less than a one percent failure rate. The other choices have a nine percent, six percent, and twenty-eight percent failure rates, respectively.

Made in the USA
Columbia, SC
02 October 2021